the
DIABETES
HANDBOOK

Ruth E. Lundstrom, MSN, NP, CDE
Aldo A. Rossini, MD

JONES AND BARTLETT PUBLISHERS
Sudbury, Massachusetts
BOSTON   TORONTO   LONDON   SINGAPORE

World Headquarters
Jones and Bartlett
Publishers
40 Tall Pine Drive
Sudbury, MA 01776
info@jbpub.com
www.jbpub.com

Jones and Bartlett
Publishers Canada
2406 Nikanna Road
Mississauga, ON L5C
2W6
CANADA

Jones and Bartlett
Publishers International
Barb House, Barb Mews
London W6 7PA
UK

Library of Congress Cataloging-in-Publication Data

Lundstrom, Ruth, 1943-
    The diabetes handbook / Ruth Lundstrom, Aldo A. Rossini.
        p. cm.
    ISBN 0-7637-2386-X
    1. Diabetes—Popular works.   2. Diabetes—Handbooks, manuals, etc.
I. Rossini, Aldo A. II. Title.
    RC660.4.L86 2003
    616.4'62—dc22

                                                        2003016741

The authors, editor, and publisher have made every effort to provide accurate information. However, they are not responsible for errors, omissions, or any outcomes related to the use of the contents of this book and take no responsibility for the use of the products described. Treatments and side effects described in this book may not be applicable to all patients; likewise, some patients may require a dose or experience a side effect that is not described herein. The reader should confer with his or her own physician regarding specific treatments and side effects. Drugs and medical devices are discussed that may have limited availability controlled by the Food and Drug Administration (FDA) for use only in a research study or clinical trial. The drug information presented has been derived from reference sources, recently published data, and pharmaceutical research data. Research, clinical practice, and government regulations often change the accepted standard in this field. When consideration is being given to use of any drug in the clinical setting, the healthcare provider or reader is responsible for determining FDA status of the drug, reading the package insert, reviewing prescribing information for the most up-to-date recommendations on dose, precautions, and contraindications, and determining the appropriate usage for the product. This is especially important in the case of drugs that are new or seldom used.

Production Credits:
Acquisitions Editor: Christopher Davis
Production Editor: Elizabeth Platt
Illustrations: Ursula Wisniewski
Additional Art: ANCOart, Inc.
Cover Design: Kristin Ohlin
Text Design: Anne Spencer
Manufacturing Buyer: Therese Bräuer
Composition: Interactive Composition Corporation
Printing and Binding: Malloy, Inc.
Cover Printer: Malloy, Inc.

Printed in the United States of America
07 06 05 04 03   10 9 8 7 6 5 4 3 2 1

Contents

CHAPTER 4 Type 2 Diabetes   51

CHAPTER 5 Monitoring   61

CHAPTER 6 Nutrition   75

CHAPTER 7 Exercise and Activity   97

CHAPTER 8 Insulin   119

CHAPTER 9 Oral Medications 155

CHAPTER 10 Sick Day Management 161

CHAPTER 11 Foot Care, Skin, and Dental Hygiene 171

CHAPTER 12 Complications   183

CHAPTER 13 Diabetes and the Family   197

CHAPTER 14 Traveling   221

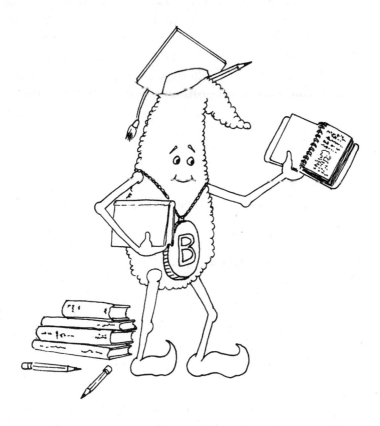

Introduction

You have diabetes, and thus, you likely have a lot of questions: Why me? Can I still lead a normal life? How will I take care of myself?

It's time to begin learning about diabetes and how to live with it. Your education about diabetes is similar to going back to school. This time, however, you won't be studying math, science, history, or Latin, although you will learn

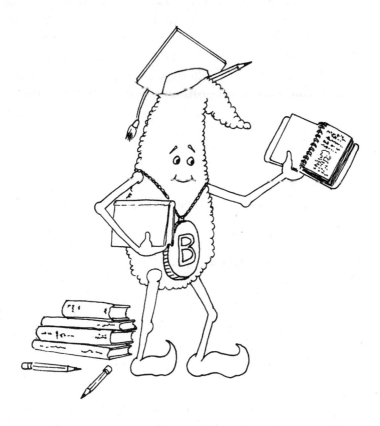

something about each of these as they relate to diabetes. You'll be studying diabetes—what causes it, how you can adapt your lifestyle to it, and how to care for yourself. You'll be studying life—**your** life—with diabetes. The more that you know about diabetes and about your self-management plan, the less frightened you will be. Knowledge, understanding, and the support of family, friends, and your healthcare team will empower you. This handbook is your basic text. It holds the answers to many of your questions, and it's filled with advice to help you manage your diabetes and still do almost everything that you've done before. Because well-meaning people may offer stories, opinions, and advice that could be confusing, you should get the facts from your healthcare providers and from Professor B, who is your instructor for this course. He's shaped like the pancreas and wears the letter B to remind you about the **beta cells** in the pancreas, where insulin is produced in people who do not have diabetes. In people with diabetes, the beta cells either malfunction or are destroyed.

Here's what you'll find in this book:

- **Chapter 1: What Is Diabetes?**—This contains diabetes definitions, causes, and history, as well as an overview of insulin, the pancreas, and kidney functioning.

- **Chapter 2: Coping with Diabetes**—This offers practical advice for accepting your diabetes emotionally and living with it day to day. Plus, you'll get "your guide to better diabetes care."

- **Chapter 3: Type 1 Diabetes Mellitus**—This is a description of Type 1 diabetes. If you've been diagnosed with this type of diabetes, you'll want to pay special attention to this chapter.

- **Chapter 4: Type 2 Diabetes Mellitus**—This is a description of Type 2 diabetes. If you've been diagnosed with this type of diabetes, you'll want to pay special attention to this chapter.

- **Chapter 5: Monitoring**—This explains how to keep track of your blood sugar level to help control your diabetes. It's important that you read this chapter no matter which kind of diabetes you have.

- **Chapter 6: Nutrition**—This contains information that everyone with diabetes needs to understand in order to control diabetes. You'll learn how to plan meals at home or when dining out.

- **Chapter 7: Exercise and Activity**—This contains advice on exercise programs for people with diabetes. Whether you have Type 1 or Type 2 diabetes, exercise can help to keep you healthy.

- **Chapter 8: Insulin**—This teaches you about the types of insulin, how to buy and store insulin, how to inject insulin, and how to avoid and treat insulin reactions. If you're not injecting insulin, you can skip this chapter.

- **Chapter 9: Oral Medications**—This contains information for people who take diabetes pills. If you do not take diabetes pills, you can skip this chapter.

- **Chapter 10: Sick Day Management**—This is a guide to diabetes control during illness. Read this chapter carefully so that you know how to cope with illness **before** you get sick.

- **Chapter 11: Skin and Foot Care**—This lists easy things that you can do to avoid some of the most commonly experienced problems related to diabetes.

- **Chapter 12: Complications**—This describes complications that are associated with diabetes and offers advice on how to avoid them.

- **Chapter 13: Diabetes and the Family**—This presents information and advice for families who are coping with diabetes. Part I of this chapter explains the special concerns of pregnant women with diabetes. Part II offers advice to parents of children with diabetes. Part III gives information for school personnel who have contact with students who have diabetes. Part IV gives information on how to support a family member with diabetes.

- **Chapter 14: Traveling**—This offers tips that help to ensure safe, healthy trips for people with diabetes.

- **Chapter 15: Research**—This highlights current research activities into the causes and prevention of and potential treatments for diabetes.

These chapters are constructed to help you learn about diabetes and also to make information available when you need it. Some of the chapters end with a series of questions and answers that clarify information further. Several chapters list products for people with diabetes or refer to other publications on diabetes. Your healthcare provider can advise you about products and publications as well. Read this book carefully. Take notes if it helps you to learn. Be sure to write the questions that you may have as you are reading, and go over them with your diabetes educator. The more you know about diabetes, the better control you will achieve. Better control means good health and a long life.

What Is Diabetes?

Let's start with the origins of diabetes.

Origins

The medical name for diabetes, **diabetes mellitus,** comes from words with Greek and Latin roots. **Diabetes** comes from a Greek word that means **to siphon.** The most obvious sign of diabetes is excessive urination. Water passes through the body of a person with diabetes as if it were being siphoned from the mouth through the urinary system and out of the body.

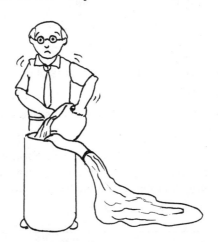

Mellitus comes from a Latin word that means **sweet like honey.** The urine of a person with diabetes contains extra sugar (glucose). In 1679, a physician tasted the urine of a person with diabetes and described it as sweet like honey.

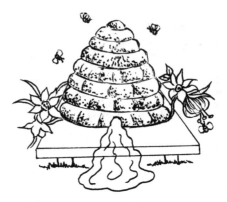

Anyone can get diabetes. In fact, 16 million Americans from all walks of life have diabetes, including famous entertainers, athletes, and political leaders. Although they must carefully balance their food, exercise, and medication, most people with diabetes lead full, active lives.

A History of Diabetes	
1500 BC	Ebers Papyrus first described diabetes.
400 BC	Susruta recorded diabetes symptoms and classified types of diabetes. Charaka refined this work in 6 AD.
10 AD	Celsus developed a clinical description of diabetes.
20 AD	Aretaeus coined the term diabetes.
1869	Langerhans described clusters of cells (islets) in the pancreas.
1889	von Mering and Minkowski observed that diabetes develops when an animal's pancreas is removed.
1921	Banting and Best obtained and purified islets of Langerhans from an animal's pancreas, injected the material (insulin) into a diabetic animal, and found a fall in blood sugar level.

The Role of Insulin

Insulin, a hormone that is produced in the pancreas, regulates the amount of sugar in the blood. In those with diabetes, the pancreas produces no insulin, not enough insulin to control blood sugar, or defective insulin. To understand how this affects you, you need to understand more about how insulin works in your body.

Think of each of the billions of cells in your body as a tiny machine. Like all machines, cells need fuel. The foods that you eat are made up of three main nutrients: carbohydrates, proteins, and fats, which are broken down to provide fuel for the cells. **The main fuel used by the cells is called glucose, a simple sugar.** Glucose is a carbohydrate. Although carbohydrates are the main source of glucose, protein also makes some glucose—but at much lesser quantities and much slower rates.

Glucose enters your cells through **receptors,** which are sites on cells that accept insulin and allow glucose to enter. Once inside, glucose can be used as fuel, but glucose has difficulty entering your cells without insulin. Think of insulin as the funnel that allows glucose (sugar) to pass through the receptors into your cells.

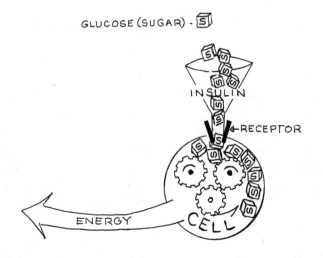

Excess glucose is stored in the liver and muscles in a form called **glycogen.** Between meals, when your blood sugar is low and your cells need fuel, the liver glycogen is released to form glucose. When the liver and muscle cells are full of glycogen, your body will convert the rest of the glucose to fat for long-term storage.

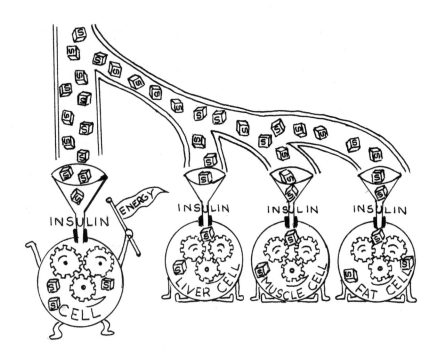

Pancreas, Islets of Langerhans, and Beta Cells

The **pancreas** is located in the abdomen, behind the stomach, and is attached to the small intestine and the spleen. Inside the pancreas are small clusters of cells called **Islets of Langerhans.** Within the islets, the majority of the cells are **beta cells,** which produce insulin.

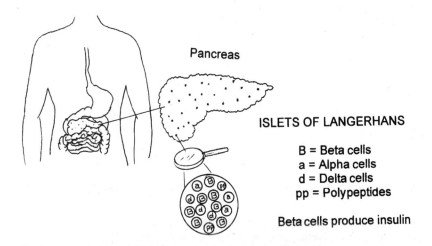

Pancreas

ISLETS OF LANGERHANS

B = Beta cells
a = Alpha cells
d = Delta cells
pp = Polypeptides

Beta cells produce insulin

In people who do not have diabetes, glucose in the blood stimulates production of insulin in the beta cells.

Beta cells "measure" blood glucose levels constantly and deliver the required amount of insulin to funnel glucose into cells. This keeps blood sugar in the normal range of 60 to 110 mg.

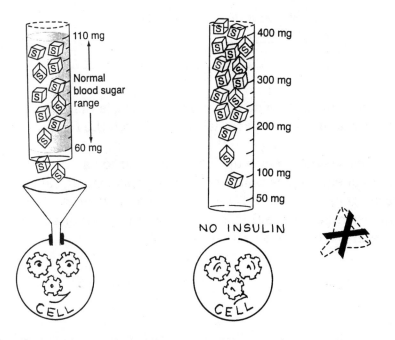

When there is little or no insulin in the body or when insulin is not working properly, glucose has difficulty entering your cells. Also, when there is not enough insulin, excess glucose cannot be stored in the liver and muscle tissue. Instead, glucose accumulates in your blood. This high concentration of glucose in the blood is called **hyperglycemia** or high blood sugar.

Where Does Blood Sugar Come From?

Everyone knows that eating sugar can put sugar into the blood. As mentioned before, all carbohydrate foods become sugar, and more than half of the protein that we eat turns to sugar also. Every person with diabetes knows that one of the key parts of controlling blood sugar is paying attention to nutrition (see Chapter 6).

FOOD GROUPS	SUGAR CONVERSION
CARBOHYDRATES	100%
PROTEINS	60%
FATS	0%

What many people do not know, however, is that not all of the sugar in the blood comes directly from the food that we eat. Because sugar in the blood is so important to our bodies, we have a backup source of sugar to use when we are not eating. The main source is stores of sugar, called **glycogen,** in the liver. The liver is like a big factory that makes many of the things that we need to live, one of which is blood sugar (**glucose**).

To understand this whole process, let's look at how our bodies process food.

When we eat, the food is broken down in our gut into small units that we can absorb. Some is used for energy, some to build and repair the body, and some is converted into storage units for later use. **Carbohydrate** foods (bread, pasta, rice, fruits, etc.) enter the stomach and are broken down in the gut into glucose. Glucose gets absorbed into the bloodstream and is distributed to the brain and other organs. Some of the glucose goes to the liver and is changed to glycogen for storage.

Protein foods (meat, fish, poultry, eggs, etc.) enter the stomach and are broken down in the gut to amino acids and glucose. **Amino acid**s are the building blocks for the body. The amino acids are picked up in the bloodstream and transported to the liver, where they are converted to glycogen for storage.

During the night when we sleep and are not eating, the liver breaks down the glycogen stores and releases it as glucose into the blood stream. This is an essential process to support a normal glucose level of 60 to 110 mg. Fat and muscle cells may also be converted to glucose during longer periods without food. **Insulin** regulates this entire process.

If you skip breakfast, the liver may actually make new sugar for you to use. It makes this new sugar from proteins that are taken away from your muscles. Without adequate insulin, this process is unregulated, and high blood sugars may occur even when one is not eating.

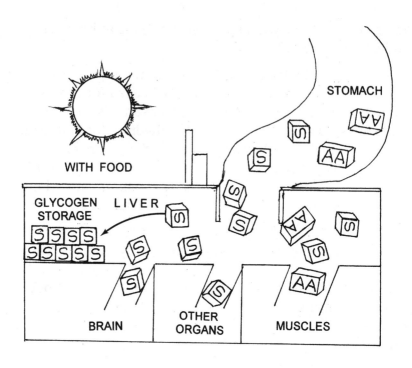

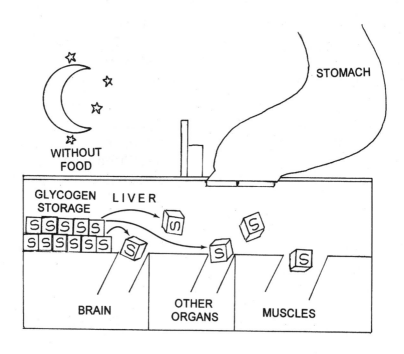

Diabetes Symptoms

People with diabetes experience different symptoms. You may experience all, some, or none of the following:

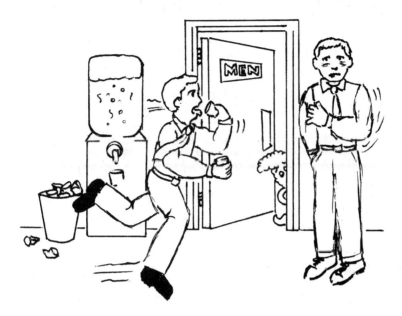

- Frequent urination (even at night).
- Excessive thirst.
- Tiredness and weakness.
- Irritability.
- Weight loss.
- Constant hunger.
- Blurry eyesight.
- Itchy skin.
- Dry skin.
- Cuts that heal slowly.
- Skin infections.
- Numbness or tingling in feet.

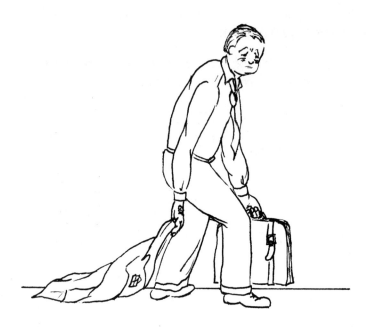

Causes of Symptoms

When blood glucose rises above a certain level, it is removed from the body in urine. Picture the kidney as a dam: When there is too much glucose in the blood, the excess "spills" out. The maximum blood glucose level reached before sugar spills is called the kidney threshold (usually approximately 180 mg).

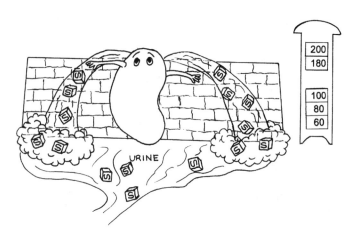

Some people with long-term diabetes or kidney disease can have a very high kidney threshold. Sugar will not "spill" into the urine until the blood sugar is very high. Dehydration also causes a high kidney threshold.

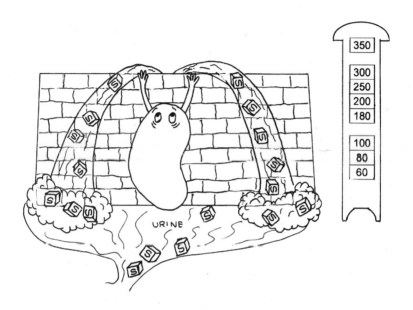

Glucose cannot be passed out of the body alone. Sugar sucks up water so that it can "flow" from the body, resulting in **polyuria** or **excessive urination**. People with excess glucose in their blood, as in uncontrolled diabetes, make frequent trips to the bathroom. These people also have sugar in their urine, medically termed **glycosuria**.

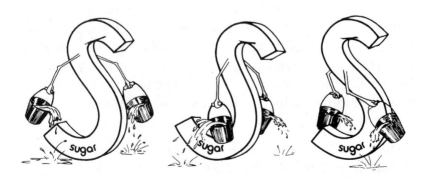

A loss of water through urination triggers the brain to send a message of thirst. This results in a condition called **polydipsia,** or **excessive thirst.** This symptom is not always pronounced, however; you may notice nothing more than a dry mouth.

Excessive urination can result in **dehydration,** leading to dry skin. Fluctuations in the amount of glucose and water in the lenses in your eyes during periods of fluctuating blood sugar can cause **blurred vision.** When there is no insulin to funnel glucose into the body's cells or when the insulin funnel is not working to pass glucose sugar through the receptors, the cells get no fuel and thus starve.

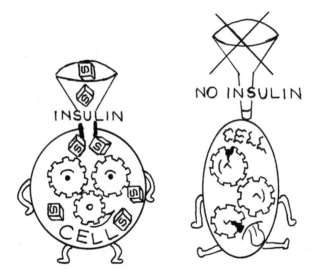

This triggers the brain to send a message of hunger, resulting in **polyphagia** or excessive hunger. Because the glucose that should be fueling your cells is flowing out in urine, the cells cannot produce energy, and without energy, you may feel weak or tired. Weight loss may occur in people whose bodies produce no insulin because without insulin, no fuel enters their cells.

Insulin also works to keep fuels inside of the cells. When insulin is low, the body breaks down the fuels, and rapid weight loss results. The breakdown of fat cells forms fatty acids, which pass through the liver to form **ketones,** which are excreted in the urine. The medical term for ketones in the urine is **ketonuria.**

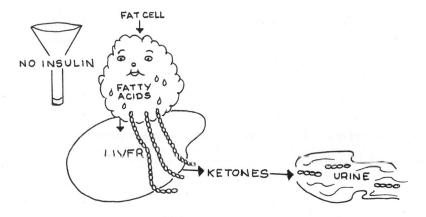

Skin infections sometimes occur because excess sugar in the blood suppresses the natural defense mechanisms (e.g., the action of white blood cells). Sugar is an excellent food in which bacteria and fungi grow. An overgrowth of bacteria worsens the infection.

Numbness and tingling in feet and **night leg cramps** may result from nerve damage and changes in the nerves that prolonged high glucose levels cause.

Types of Diabetes

Almost all people with diabetes have one of two major types (the other types are mentioned later in Chapter 1): Type 1 and Type 2. Approximately 10% have Type 1 diabetes mellitus, in which their bodies produce **no** insulin. When diagnosed, most people with Type 1 diabetes are under 25 and are usually thin. Symptoms are often pronounced and come on suddenly. Because their bodies produce no insulin, people with Type 1 diabetes must obtain insulin through injection. If you've been diagnosed with Type 1 diabetes, you'll want to pay special attention to Chapter 3.

Approximately 85% of persons with diabetes have Type 2 diabetes mellitus. Their bodies have become resistant to the action of insulin. Thus, although they produce some insulin, it isn't enough or it doesn't work properly to funnel glucose through the receptors into their cells. When diagnosed, most people with Type 2 diabetes are over 35 and are usually overweight. Recently, there has been an increase in the number of children and young adults who are diagnosed with Type 2 diabetes. Symptoms are usually not pronounced and appear over a long period of time. Often the diagnosis of diabetes is made at a routine visit to the doctor. Type 2 diabetes can sometimes be controlled with a carefully planned diet and exercise, but oral medications or insulin injections may be necessary. If you have Type 2 diabetes, you can find information in Chapter 4.

This table highlights some of the differences between Type 1 and Type 2 diabetes.

	Type 1	Type 2
Age at onset	Usually under 25 years old	Usually over 40 years old
Body weight	Thin/normal weight	Usually overweight
Symptoms	Appear suddenly	Appear slowly
Insulin produced	None	Too little
Insulin required	Requires insulin	May require insulin
Previously called names	Juvenile diabetes, insulin dependent	Adult-onset diabetes, noninsulin dependent

How Is Diabetes Diagnosed?

Both Type 1 and Type 2 diabetes are diagnosed when you have a consistent fasting blood sugar that is over 126 mg/dl or a casual blood sugar over 200 mg/dl. A diagnosis of diabetes can also be established when symptoms of diabetes are present with one blood sugar over 200 mg/dl.

Other Types of Diabetes

People whose blood contains more glucose than normal, but less than occurs in diabetes, may be diagnosed with a condition called **impaired fasting glucose** (fasting blood sugar over 110 mg/dl but not over 126 mg/dl). Some women experience a rise in their blood glucose level during pregnancy. These women have a condition called **gestational diabetes mellitus.** Their blood glucose levels usually return to normal after their babies are born. Other types of diabetes may occur as a result of diseases of the pancreas or the endocrine (gland) system, genetic disorders, or exposure to chemical agents, called **secondary diabetes mellitus.**

Causes of Diabetes

Heredity and obesity are two important factors in the development of diabetes:

Heredity: If you have a parent, grandparent, brother, or sister, or even a cousin who has diabetes, you are more likely to develop diabetes yourself. There is an approximately 2% to 7% risk of developing Type 1 diabetes if your mother or father or a sibling has Type 1 diabetes. There is a higher risk (up to 90%) of developing Type 2 diabetes if your parent or siblings have Type 2 diabetes and you are overweight.

Excess weight is an important factor in diabetes. Eighty percent of people with Type 2 diabetes are overweight when diagnosed. Losing weight won't cure diabetes, but it can help to reduce or even eliminate some of the symptoms.

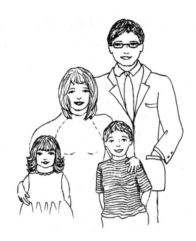

Obesity: Eighty percent of people with Type 2 diabetes are overweight when diagnosed. Obesity makes it difficult to produce enough insulin to control blood sugars. Diabetes symptoms disappear in many of these obese patients when they lose weight.

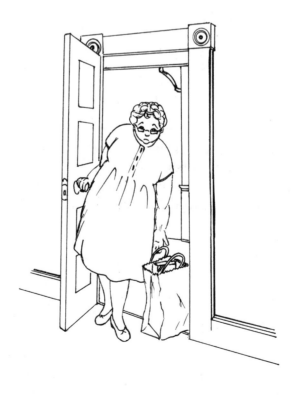

Other Factors That Can Cause or Trigger Diabetes

- *Age:* As people age, their bodies may have fewer insulin-producing beta cells.

- *Viruses:* Certain viruses may destroy beta cells or may trigger the immune system to destroy beta cells in susceptible people.

- *Faulty immune system:* Scientists now believe that there is not one cause of diabetes but multiple factors that may trigger the immune system to destroy beta cells.

- *Physical trauma:* An accident or injury may destroy the pancreas, where insulin is normally produced.

- *Drugs:* Drugs prescribed for another condition may un-mask diabetes by causing insulin resistance or destroying beta cells.

- *Stress:* Hormones released during periods of stress, such as an acute illness or surgery, may decrease the action of insulin.

- *Pregnancy:* Hormones produced during pregnancy may decrease the action of insulin.

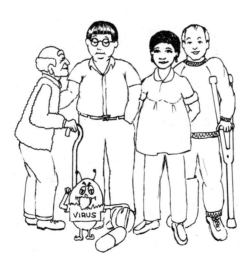

Why Is Controlling Diabetes Important?

Here are four reasons:

1. To feel well and be free of the symptoms of diabetes.
2. To have energy to pursue education, work, recreation, and activities.
3. To minimize complications.
4. To live a normal life span.

Control of diabetes means balancing the amounts of sugar and insulin in your blood. To achieve this balance, your healthcare provider will help you develop a plan for food, exercise, and possibly insulin injections or oral medications. Sticking to your plan helps to keep you healthy and greatly reduces your risk of developing diabetes complications.

People with diabetes are at risk for a variety of complications over time. Healthcare providers all agree that tight control of blood sugar makes complications less likely. This was shown clearly by two major studies conducted in the United States and Europe. Control of blood sugar is the best way to minimize the risk of complications.

If you're feeling fine, you may wonder whether you really have to follow your healthcare provider's advice. Remember that not everyone who has diabetes experiences the same (or any) symptoms. Even if you notice no symptoms, you still have diabetes, and keeping your blood glucose in control is still important because high blood sugar is toxic for your body. You may adapt to high blood sugars, giving you a false sense of feeling fine. However, over time, it can result in damage to your blood vessels, kidneys, eyes, and nerves. Remember that the closer your blood glucose level is to normal, the healthier your body will be.

Don't let yourself believe that a lack of symptoms means you don't still need to control your blood glucose levels. Over time, the high blood glucose levels in your body can result in damage to your blood vessels, kidneys, eyes, and nerves. Remember that the closer your blood glucose level is to normal, the healthier your body will be.

Can Diabetes Be Cured?

There are no easy cures for most cases of diabetes. Some people with diabetes can be cured by a pancreas transplant or by transplanting insulin-producing cells, but there are significant risks associated with the surgery and with the immunosuppression drugs that need to be taken. Even if diabetes cannot be easily cured, it can be controlled.

Resources

Keep informed about diabetes. The more you know, the better you will be able to take care of yourself. By joining the organizations listed here, you will gain access to a network that can provide the latest information on diabetes research and treatment.

- American Diabetes Association
  1600 Duke Street
  Alexandria, VA 22314
  1-800-237-3472
  Website: www.diabetes.org

- General Membership
  P.O. Box 2055
  Harlan, IA 51593–0238
  1-800-806-7801
  (The membership fee includes subscription to *Diabetes Forecast* magazine.)

Many local chapters of the American Diabetes Association exist. Contact the American Diabetes Association for their list of local affiliations.

- Juvenile Diabetes Foundation International
  120 Wall Street, 19th Floor
  New York, NY 10005-4001
  1-212-785-9595
  Website: www.jdfcure.org
  (The membership fee includes subscription to *Countdown* magazine.)

Many local chapters of the Juvenile Diabetes Foundation exist (contact the Juvenile Diabetes Foundation for a list of their local affiliates).

- Diabetes Self-Management
  P.O. Box 51125
  Boulder, CO 80321–1125

- Diabetes in the News
  P.O. Box 3105
  Elkhart, IN 46515

- National Diabetes
  Information
  Clearing House
  One Information Way
  Bethesda, MD 20892–3560
  1-301-654-3327
  E-mail: ndic@aerie.com

Finally, you may want to consult some of the growing number of online resources that are about diabetes. The list is expanding and is frequently being updated. This handbook probably won't answer all of the questions that you have about diabetes. In several chapters, you'll find references to other books that you may want to read for more information.

Purchase any of the following books online from the American Diabetes Association bookstore (www.store.diabetes.org or phone at 1-800-232-6723).

- *The Diabetic Problem Solver: Quick Answers to Your Questions about Treatment and Self-Care.* Nancy Touchette, PhD.

- *Diabetes A to Z*, 4th ed. American Diabetes Association.

- *Getting a Grip on Diabetes: Quick Tips and Techniques for Kids and Teens.* Nasmyth-Loy & Nasmyth-Loy.

- *I Am Loved: True Stories of True Love from People Like You.* Edited by Rich Davis and Barnett Helzberg.

- *American Diabetes Association Complete Guide to Diabetes,* 2nd ed. American Diabetes Association.

CHAPTER 2

Coping with Diabetes

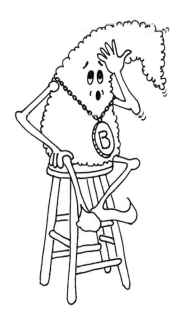

How do you cope with life's problems or with stress when you're confronted by a challenge? Do you gather all of the available information? Do you get help from others? Do you express or hide your feelings or hope that the problem will go away? It's important to pay attention to your feelings and to understand that they are normal. Developing a positive attitude and confidence in your ability to manage your diabetes will set a course for health and happiness.

Coping with Psychological Aspects of Diabetes

Some people don't believe that they have diabetes and thus don't see why they need to follow a diabetes care plan. Others understand that they have diabetes but still do not follow their care plans. Both of these responses are forms of **denial.** It can take time to overcome denial, but the sooner that you accept your diagnosis and begin learning about diabetes, the sooner you'll achieve independence and good health.

Although it is normal for people who are diagnosed with diabetes to experience **anger,** you won't help yourself by remaining angry and hostile. Try talking and expressing these feelings to family members, friends, or others with diabetes. Consider directing the energy from the anger to do something positive (e.g., volunteering or fund raising for diabetes organizations).

Maybe you feel **guilty** and think that you did something to cause your diabetes. Was it all of the candy that you ate? Was it binge eating? Are you being punished for something bad that you have done? **NO!** None of these cause diabetes. If they did, almost everyone would have it. Whenever you feel that diabetes is a punishment for something that you did, review the causes of diabetes in Chapter 1 to remind yourself that diabetes can happen to anyone.

Depression can be a serious problem for people with diabetes. Symptoms of depression include feelings of helplessness or hopelessness, loneliness, a lack of self-esteem, fatigue, irritability, and changes in sleep patterns or eating habits. If you experience any of these symptoms, get help. Your healthcare provider can refer you to counselors who have experience in helping people with diabetes and depression. Many people with diabetes will experience a time of **grieving.** After first being diagnosed with diabetes or when a complication occurs, it is normal to grieve over the loss of your healthy self. With time and support from family, healthcare providers, religious leaders, and friends, you will be able to resolve this grief.

One of the most difficult things that you will face is the knowledge that even if you follow your diabetes care plan completely, you may not achieve perfect control. Following your regimen is no guarantee that you will be healthy forever. Then why bother? Because working at good control will help you to feel better, both physically and emotionally. You'll feel better when you're doing everything possible to stay well. The only way to reduce your risk of complications is to keep good control of your diabetes. Take one day at a time and one step at a time.

Your Own Coping Skills

Diabetes is a serious condition that requires your own strength, energy, and attention, as well as the support of your friends and family. Commit yourself to taking responsibility for your self-management, following your regime, and learning as much as you can about your diabetes.

How do you feel about having diabetes? Do you see it as a daily challenge—one that requires your own strength, energy, and attention, as well as the support of your friends and family? If so, you're probably coping well with your diabetes, and you understand that diabetes is a serious condition and are optimistic about your treatment plan. You're committed to taking responsibility for your self-management, following your regime, and learning as much as you can about your diabetes. You trust your healthcare team and feel free to participate in decisions about your diabetes care plan. Coping also includes being assertive to make sure that you have time to check your blood sugar, get meals when you need them, and get a full exam from your healthcare provider. Your attitude is positive.

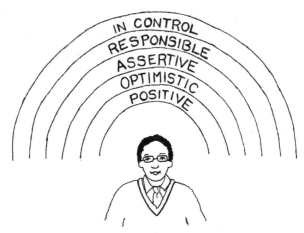

IN CONTROL
RESPONSIBLE
ASSERTIVE
OPTIMISTIC
POSITIVE

On the other hand, if you believe that diabetes isn't a serious condition, that your care plan is impossible to follow, or that your treatment won't work, then you're not coping well. Maybe you feel that it's your doctor's responsibility to keep you well, that you can't change your lifestyle to fit your diabetes regimen, that you have no time for medical appointments, or that you can't depend on family and friends for support. These are all negative coping responses.

If you feel that you're not coping well with diabetes, ask yourself for the reasons. Do you think you are not strong enough, smart enough, or educated enough to take responsibility for your self-management? Are you afraid that you can't afford diabetes supplies? Your first step is to seek out trustworthy healthcare professionals who will work as team members. It takes courage and hope to get involved in your own care, but it's worth the effort. Each person reacts to diabetes in a unique way.

Tips for Living Well with Diabetes

TIPS FOR LIVING WELL WITH DIABETES

ACCEPT and make CHANGES
LEARN all you can
Take RESPONSIBILITY
Set GOALS
SHARE your feelings
Keep POSITIVE
Be FLEXIBLE
CONNECT with a team
GET HELP!

- Accept the fact that you have diabetes and that you will need to make some changes in your lifestyle.

- Learn all that you can about your diabetes and its treatment.

- Take responsibility for diabetes self-management.

- Set goals and objectives, but remember that it takes time.

- Share your feelings with family and friends and help them learn about diabetes.

- Keep a positive attitude.

- Be flexible and learn to fit diabetes into your life.

- Find a healthcare team (possibly a doctor, a nurse, a practitioner, a registered nurse, a registered dietitian, a certified diabetes educator, a psychologist, a social worker, a pharmacist, an exercise physiologist, and a podiatrist) with whom you connect.
- Get help to change behaviors that are harmful to your diabetes plan of care.
- Live life to its fullest.

Remember that life is 10% of what happens to you and 90% of how you respond.

Roles and Rights

You and your healthcare team have a responsibility to help you to stay in the best health possible. You will work with your healthcare team to select goals and to make some changes. Your healthcare team will provide the following:

1. Diabetes self-management education, which includes information about the following:

   - Diabetes process.
   - Nutrition management.
   - Physical activity and exercise.
   - Medications (pills and insulin).
   - Blood sugar monitoring.
   - Acute complications (problems with low and high blood sugars).
   - Chronic complications (problems with eyes, kidneys, nerves, blood vessels, heart, and feet).
   - Goal setting and problem solving.
   - Healthy coping behaviors.
   - Pregnancy and gestational diabetes.

2. A yearly physical exam, which includes the following:

   - Blood tests for hemoglobin A1C, thyroid, kidney function, and lipid profile (cholesterol).

- A dilated eye exam (usually done by an ophthalmologist).
- A review of your risk factors for heart disease (weight, exercise, and smoking).
- A foot exam for neuropathy and circulation.

3. Brief physical exams every 3 to 6 months, which may include the following:

- Hemoglobin A1c.
- Weight.
- Feet check.
- Blood pressure.

4. Periodic visits, which should include the following:

- A review of your blood sugar tests, weight, blood pressure, and goals.
- A discussion about your progress and a question-answering period.
- Help with problem solving and any special situations that arise.
- Evaluation of your success.
- Referrals to specialists when necessary.

Your role includes these items:

- Learning and practicing self-management.
- Examining your feet daily.
- Following a healthy lifestyle of selecting nutritious food, maintaining a healthy weight, getting regular exercise, and avoiding smoking.
- Knowing when to contact your healthcare team.
- Keeping your appointments.
- Talking to your family and friends about your needs as a person with diabetes.

Coping with the Social Aspects of Diabetes

 Diabetes is a condition covered by state and federal antidiscrimination laws. You can't legally be fired because of your diabetes, nor can an employer deny you a job for which you're qualified.

Job discrimination is against the law, but it happens. For example, some employers who have had bad experiences with employees with diabetes may be reluctant to hire you. All states have antidiscrimination statutes. To find out about the relevant laws in your state, contact the state commission on human or civil rights, the office of fair employment, or the Department of Labor. People with diabetes cannot join the armed forces, hold commercial pilot's licenses, or join the FBI. In some states, they cannot join police forces, but this policy has been challenged and overturned in some states. Federal Occupational Safety and Health Administration guidelines limit the types of machinery that can be operated by people with diabetes.

The American Diabetes Association advocates for case-by-case determination of employment eligibility. The American Diabetes Association's position is that "any person [with diabetes] should be able to accept any employment for which he or she is individually qualified." Your local American Diabetes Association affiliate can provide information about the American Diabetes Association's Attorney's Network, a group of lawyers who are experienced in helping people with diabetes. You can also contact the local bar association for referrals to lawyers with experience in employment discrimination cases. Help yourself. Don't accept a job that will conflict with your diabetes care plan. Seek employment in which you will be allowed time away for your regular checkups and in which a good health plan is offered. Your state vocational rehabilitation office can assist with vocational counseling, job placement, and retraining.

Remember that you're not "a diabetic." You're a person with diabetes.

Driver's Licenses

Most states require a doctor's certification that a person with diabetes is in good control before granting a driver's license. Bring a note from your doctor when you apply for or renew your license. It is a privilege for you to drive a car— not a right. It is your responsibility to maintain this privilege.

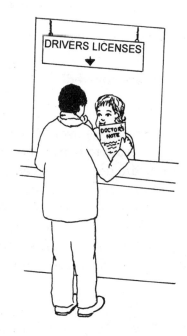

Health Insurance

Health insurance is a must for people with diabetes. Supplies and medication are expensive even if covered by insurance, as they often require a co-payment. The best deal is health insurance that employers offer because the company absorbs part of the cost.

Many types of insurance may be offered if you are with a large company, whereas only one type may be offered if you or your spouse works for a small company. The types of insurance include PPOs, HMO-managed care, and fee for services.

These questions should be considered before choosing or changing insurance:

- Are your doctors (primary care and diabetes specialist) listed on the plan?
- Are diabetes visits and diabetes education covered?
- Would your medications, supplies, and durable medical equipment be covered?
- Which hospitals can you use?
- What other services are covered?
- What are the limitations?

Medicare is available for people over 65, for those who are disabled and who are unable to work, and for those with a very low income. Medicare does not cover medications, including insulin and syringes, but it does cover test strips. Many people will purchase Medigap policies, which cover gaps in the coverage. Read the complete policy to be sure that you're getting what you need before purchasing the policy. Call your local Social Security Administration office for information.

Medicaid is a federal and state assistance program for very low-income people. Because eligibility varies from state to state, you should call your local Medicaid office for information about eligibility requirements.

Diabetes Identification

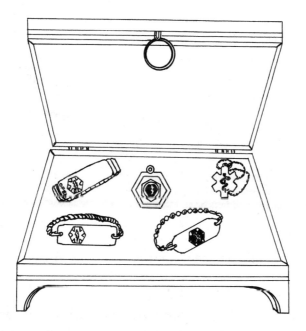

Your healthcare provider may suggest that you wear a bracelet, tag, or necklace, or that you carry a card in your wallet that identifies you as having diabetes. This is helpful in emergency situations in which you might not be able to speak to the healthcare provider who is assisting you.

Media Hype

Advertising for new diabetes drugs or non-prescription herbal preparations may not give you a complete picture of what the drug or herb does, or how it might interact with your current medications. Talk to your doctor about what you've seen or read, and discuss any medications, even over-the-counter supplements, with your doctor before you use them.

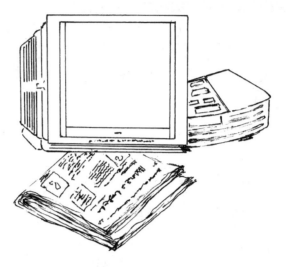

You will hear ads on the radio for drugs, see drug-promoting skits on TV, or catch an article in a magazine or flyer that are all trying to entice you to ask your healthcare provider about a new wonder drug for diabetes or diabetes complications. The ads quickly throw side effects at you to try to lessen the impact. If you have questions about any drugs that you've heard or seen advertised, discuss them with your healthcare provider, as you may already be on an equivalent medication and/or one that is working well for you.

Other ads promote herbal preparations, vitamins, and minerals that may promise an array of miracles from curing diabetes to reversing complications. The claims are not supported by good research. **Some of these over-the-counter preparations can interfere with the action of your medications and may be outright dangerous.** At the very least, you could waste time and your money. Discuss any of these preparations with your healthcare provider. If they are not harmful, then go ahead and try them. If you see no improvement in 3 to 6 months, then it is doubtful that you are getting your money's worth.

Resources

Psyching Out Diabetes: A Positive Approach to Your Negative Emotions. Richard Rubin, PhD, June Biermann, and Barbara Toohey.

Reflections on Diabetes. Published by the American Diabetes Association.

When Diabetes Hits Home. Wendy Satin Rapaport, LICSW, PsyD.

When Bad Things Happen to Good People. Rabbi Kushner.

CHAPTER 3

Type 1 Diabetes

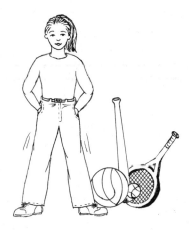

Goals for People with Type 1 Diabetes

Learning that you or your child has Type 1 diabetes can be devastating; however, you can overcome this challenge by learning how to live successfully with diabetes.

Take a Goal-Oriented Approach

- Learn how to balance food, exercise, and insulin.
- Become self-reliant and self-sufficient.
- Protect your heart, nerves, blood vessels, eyes, and kidneys by controlling your blood glucose level.
- Maintain a good body weight.
- Lead an active, productive life.
- Target normal growth and development for children.

What Causes Type 1 Diabetes?

Scientists have been trying to answer this question for many years. There are several factors that make a person susceptible to getting Type 1 diabetes:

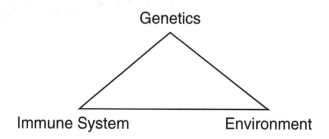

1. The following shows the relationships between genetic factors and the susceptibility or resistance to Type 1 diabetes:

   - Over 80% of new cases have no known family history of diabetes.
   - If one parent has Type 1 diabetes, the risk is 7%.
   - If a sibling has diabetes, there is a 5% to 17% risk.
   - An identical twin has a 30% to 50% risk of getting diabetes when their twin has Type 1 diabetes.

2. There are a number of environmental factors that initiate the destruction of the beta cell. Viruses (especially mumps, rubella, and Coxsackie) have been associated with this destructive process.

3. **Autoimmunity** occurs when the immune system gets misdirected to destroy healthy cells. When the beta cells in your pancreas are destroyed, they can no longer make insulin, and Type 1 diabetes occurs.

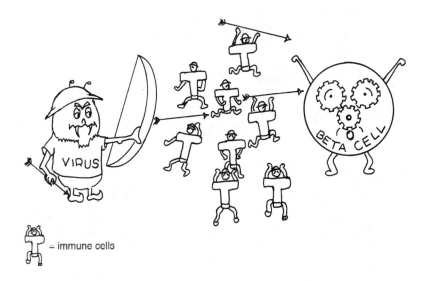

= immune cells

Symptoms of Diabetes

When you were diagnosed with Type 1 diabetes your blood sugar was probably over 300 mg, and ketones were present in your urine. You were likely very thirsty (polydipsia), passing urine frequently day (polyuria) and night (nocturia), and were very hungry (polyphagia)—eating a lot, yet losing weight. You were probably tired all of the time and may have even gotten a bad stomachache and felt air hunger. These symptoms were caused by high blood sugar and the breakdown of body fats into ketones. This happened because you had an absolute lack of insulin (see the Box, p. 44).

When you received insulin by injection, many of these symptoms went away and you thus felt better. Be aware that if these symptoms return, you are not getting enough insulin to keep you healthy.

A Special Problem: Diabetic Ketoacidosis

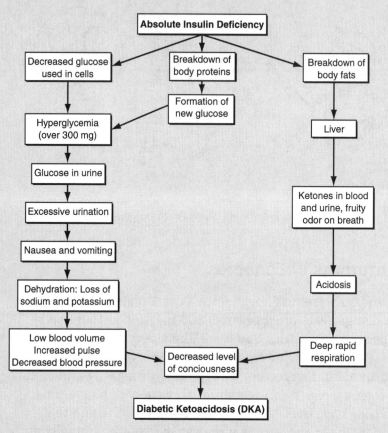

If you become ill or miss insulin doses, you will once again have the symptoms of high blood sugar (discussed previously in this chapter). Without insulin, these symptoms progress to dehydration, an increased pulse rate, and dry, flushed skin. Ketones accumulate in the blood faster than your body is able to eliminate them through the urine or exhaled breath. Breathing becomes rapid and deep, and the breath has a fruity odor. As blood sugar increases and more ketones accumulate, vomiting, stomach pains, and a decreased level of consciousness occur. Insulin and intravenous fluids can reverse this condition. You must always guard against diabetic ketoacidosis. The best way to reduce your risk of this condition is to always take your insulin, monitor your blood sugars, and follow a sick day management plan (see Chapter 10) when ill.

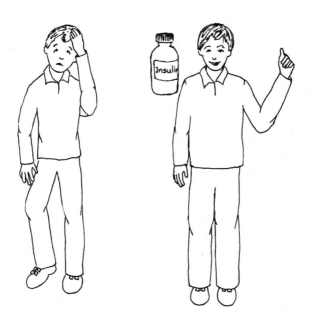

Managing Type 1 Diabetes

To control your diabetes, you and your healthcare providers need to work out a plan that includes insulin injections, exercise, and food. You will also need to learn to monitor your blood sugar level so that you will know whether your plan of insulin, exercise, and food is working.

- **Insulin injections** are necessary because your body does not produce insulin to funnel glucose into your cells. The dose of insulin will be dependent on your food intake and amount of exercise (for information on insulin, see Chapter 8).

- You and your healthcare provider will need to develop a **nutritious meal plan** to keep your diabetes in good control. Your nutrition plan provides guidelines so that you can choose from a great variety of foods (for information on nutrition, see Chapter 6).

- **Activity and exercise** improves muscle tone, increases strength and well-being, and increases the efficiency of the insulin you inject (for information on exercise programs for people with diabetes, see Chapter 7).

- To measure your success, monitor your blood sugar two to four times a day (for information on monitoring, see Chapter 5).

- A diabetes self-management education program will help you put all the pieces of the puzzle together so that you can do your best to live a long, healthy life.

Keeping in Balance

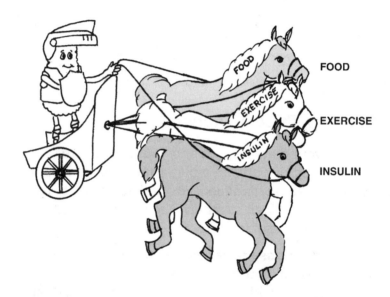

FOOD

EXERCISE

INSULIN

To stay healthy, you need to learn to balance insulin, food, and activity/exercise. The beta cells of a person without diabetes produce just the right amount of insulin to maintain a normal blood glucose level. If the person with diabetes does not eat, very little insulin is produced, but if this person eats a lot, the beta cells produce much more insulin.

Because your beta cells do not produce insulin, you must obtain it through injections. The insulin you inject controls a predefined amount of blood sugar. If you skip a meal, the insulin keeps right on working, plunging your blood sugar lower and lower. If you eat more food than the insulin you injected can handle, your blood sugar will go very high. If you exercise or are more active, you need to eat more food because exercise/activity makes insulin work more efficiently and uses more sugar for fuel.

Balancing Food, Exercise, and Insulin

- To keep in balance, stick to your meal and exercise plans, maintain your optimal weight, follow your prescribed insulin injection schedule each day, and monitor your blood sugars (if you are on a more flexible plan, your daily insulin dose may be adjusted at each meal according to your food intake and activity level).

- On days when you are more active or exercise more than usual, you need more food to keep in balance.

- On days when you eat more food than your meal plan allows, you need to increase your insulin dosage or exercise more to stay in balance.

- If you're gaining weight, you may need to increase your insulin dosage to balance the extra weight, or you may need to diet and exercise more to lose that weight. For growing children, the healthcare provider may adjust insulin to balance normal weight gains.

- If you accidentally inject more insulin than you should on a day, you must add extra food to keep in balance. Check your blood glucose every 2 to 3 hours (see Chapter 5) and eat additional snacks or meals.

In the past, you may have been taught that there was only one way to keep good diabetes control—to follow a strict diet, exercise, and insulin plan. That worked well, but it was impossible for many people to maintain day after day.

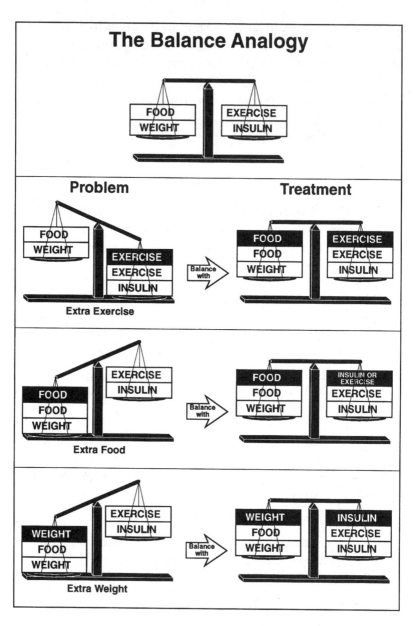

The Balance Analogy

Problem → **Treatment**

Extra Exercise

Balance with

Extra Food

Balance with

Extra Weight

Balance with

A newer approach provides much more flexibility of meals, activity, and insulin injections. It does require a little more thinking to calculate insulin doses and usually more injections. In place of strict meal plans, you may select what you want to eat, count the carbohydrates, and calculate the dose of insulin needed for the meal or snack (see Chapter 6). Correct insulin doses are calculated according to the present blood sugar and activity or exercises, which are also factored into the calculation. This plan (called intensive insulin therapy; see Chapter 8) is not difficult, but it takes practice.

Questions and Answers

Why Can't I Take Insulin by Mouth?

Insulin is a protein. If you swallow it, it is digested as smaller particles that are no longer insulin. Researchers continue to work on ways to make oral insulin a possibility.

My Friend Takes Pills for Diabetes. Why Can't I Do the Same?

The pills for diabetes work by signaling the beta cells in the pancreas to make more insulin or by helping insulin work better by lowering insulin resistance and by stopping the liver from making sugar. Your beta cells have been destroyed, and your body is producing no insulin at all; thus, the pills can't help you.

What If I Just Ignore My Diabetes?

You'll probably feel tired. You'll be thirsty and will be running to the bathroom a lot. If you get seriously out of balance and ignore these symptoms for several days, you could face the danger of a diabetic coma. If this continues for a long time, you will be at high risk for chronic diabetic complications.

What Is Brittle Diabetes?

The term "brittle" suggests that this type of diabetes is difficult to control, but when you follow guidelines designed just for you and learn how to adjust your food, activity, and insulin, this term will probably not apply.

What Is the "Honeymoon Period?"

The honeymoon period is a time shortly after diagnosis when a person seems to need very little insulin. This typically lasts 3 to 6 months, but may last for several years. During this time, diabetes is very easy to control. It's important to continue taking even small doses of insulin at this time.

What Should My Blood Sugar Be?

The normal blood sugar for people without diabetes is 60 to 110 mg/dl. Ideally, the closer to normal that you can keep your blood sugar, the better it will be for you. However, the target blood sugar is determined individually. Many other factors, such as age range and other medical conditions, are factored into the blood sugar goal.

Why Do I Feel Best When My Blood Sugar Is High and Terrible When It Gets into Normal Range?

Your body adapts to high blood sugars, giving you a false sense of well-being. Meanwhile, the excess sugar binds to proteins in your body and causes cell damage, which eventually leads to diabetic complications. At first, a normal blood sugar triggers some of the symptoms of low blood sugar, but when your body readapts to normal sugar levels, you feel great.

Resources

The Take-Charge Guide to Type 1 Diabetes. American Diabetes Association.

Understanding Insulin Dependent Diabetes. Peter Chase, MD.

Raising a Child with Diabetes. Linda Siminerio and Jean Betschart.

The Dinosaur Tamer and Other Stories for Children with Diabetes. Maria Levine Mazur, Peter Banks, and Andrew Keegan.

CHAPTER 4

Type 2 Diabetes

4

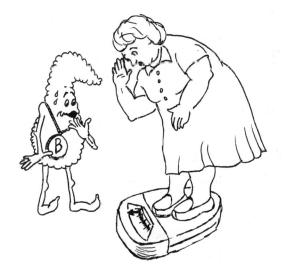

Type 2 diabetes has a slow, smoldering onset and is often diagnosed during a routine physical exam or during an illness or stressful time. Certain medications prescribed for other illnesses may unmask diabetes. Some people have Type 2 diabetes for over 10 years before they are diagnosed. Most people generally feel well or have only mild symptoms of feeling tired; thus, they are surprised to learn that they have diabetes.

After the diagnosis, don't let "doom and gloom" take over. You can make choices to follow a path that leads to health and happiness. Along the way, you will learn how nutrition, activity/exercise, and medications work together to keep your diabetes in good control. Step by step you will start to make some changes in your lifestyle that will give you power over diabetes. Don't delay—begin today.

A Goal for People with Type 2 Diabetes

People with Type 2 diabetes want to enjoy a healthy, normal life and reduce the risk of complications. These are some ways to achieve your goal:

- Learn about your diabetes and how to take care of yourself.
- Work toward your target blood sugar, blood pressure, and cholesterol levels.
- Achieve your ideal weight with a good meal plan.
- Find a personal exercise plan.
- Take special care of your feet.
- Have regular eye exams.

When you have Type 2 diabetes, your body has a "relative" deficiency of insulin.

What Is a Relative Deficiency?

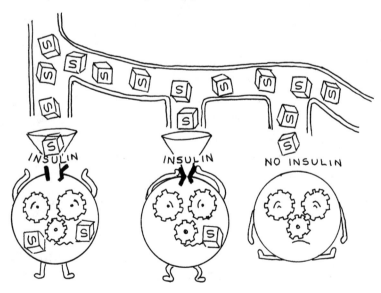

A relative deficiency occurs when the beta cells in the pancreas cannot produce enough insulin to meet the body's demands. Insulin resistance at the cell, followed by beta-cell "burnout," creates this situation. Fatigue, dry mouth, thirst, frequent urination, dry, itchy skin, slow-healing cuts or sores, more infections than usual, and numbness and tingling in toes and feet are some of the symptoms of diabetes. These symptoms may be very subtle and may go on for years without being noticed. Your healthcare provider may have diagnosed your diabetes during a routine physician exam.

What Causes Type 2 Diabetes?

There are many causes, but weight gain is most often the trigger.

1. Multiple gene defects predispose people to Type 2 diabetes.
   - Insulin resistance is caused by a genetic defect that makes insulin less effective.
   - Impaired beta cell function is caused by a genetic defect that inhibits the beta cell from making, storing, and releasing insulin.
2. Overeating leads to obesity, which is the single most important factor. A lack of exercise is also a major factor.
3. Certain medications can impair insulin release and action (resistance).
4. Without effective insulin to funnel the glucose into the body's cells, the glucose builds up in your blood (hyperglycemia).
5. When insulin levels are low, the liver breaks down glycogen (stores of sugar) and pours even more sugar into the blood.

Who Gets Type 2 Diabetes?

- One parent with diabetes increases the risk by approximately 25%, and two parents with diabetes increase the risk to more than 90%.

- Obesity causes a greater insulin demand and greater insulin resistance.

- Inactivity decreases the intake of insulin in tissues.

- The incidence increases as people age.

- Native Americans, African Americans, Asian Americans, and Hispanics have a higher prevalence.

- Mothers who have had a history of large babies (over 9 pounds) or who have had gestational diabetes are at an increased risk.

Managing Your Type 2 Diabetes

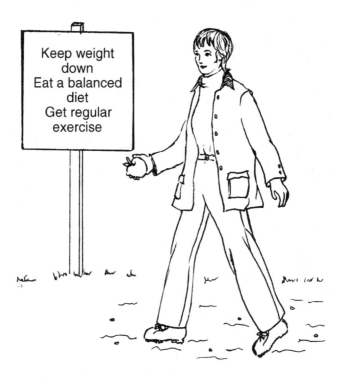

Keep weight down
Eat a balanced diet
Get regular exercise

To manage Type 2 diabetes, you need to eat right, stay active, monitor your blood sugar, take medications as prescribed, follow your healthcare provider's advice, and have regular checkups.

- **Eating right** helps you to control your weight, which is the most important factor in Type 2 diabetes control. Eat healthy foods, and if you are overweight, follow a meal plan to lose weight (for information on nutrition, see Chapter 6).

- **Staying active** with exercise burns calories to help you control your weight. Exercise also reduces insulin resistance, which helps the insulin that your body produces work more effectively (for information on exercise programs, see Chapter 7).

- **Monitoring your blood sugar** provides the information to design your diabetes care program and to remain in good control (see Chapter 5).

- **Taking medications** at the correct times each day is important (see Chapter 9).

- **Having regular checkups,** including checking your blood pressure, your feet, and your vision (yearly), is important.

- **Learning** as much as you can about your diabetes and enrolling in a diabetes self-management education program is beneficial.

Oral Agents

Your healthcare provider may prescribe oral medications or insulin (see Chapter 9). The oral medications help to stimulate your beta cells to make more insulin or to help insulin work well. Other medications reduce the amount of sugar or fat that you can absorb from the food you eat. They may be used alone or in combination.

The Weight Factor

Why is weight such an important factor in Type 2 diabetes? This scale illustrates how extra body fat affects you. Food and weight are represented by Xs, and insulin is represented by Os. In people who do not have diabetes, a balance between Xs and Os is always achieved.

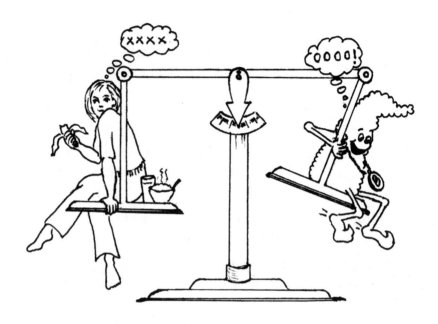

In people with Type 2 diabetes, who are usually overweight, the beta cells cannot produce enough effective insulin to maintain a balance. There are too many Xs (weight and food) for the Os (insulin) to handle. The best treatment is to decrease stored fat (Xs) to balance with the available insulin (Os)!

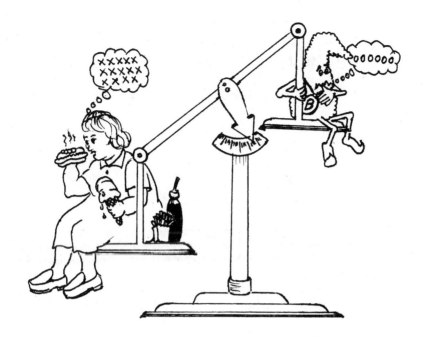

Weight Loss Tips

- Eat smaller portions (no second helpings).

- Switch to low-fat foods—eat more vegetables and fruit.

- Eat slowly.

- Serve food from the pan in which it was prepared—don't overload your plate.

- Pay attention to what you are eating. Don't let TV distract you.

- Don't skip meals, as this may cause you to overeat at the next meal.

- Store food out of sight.

- Give yourself permission to leave food on the plate—you don't have to clean the plate.

A Special Problem: Hyperosmolar Hyperglycemic Syndrome

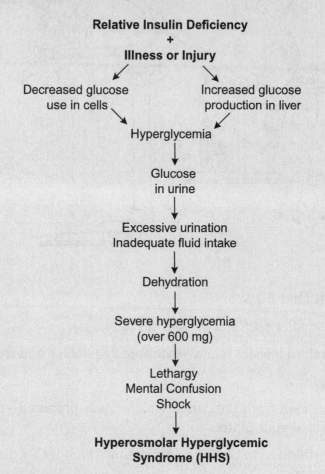

Relative Insulin Deficiency
+
Illness or Injury

Decreased glucose
use in cells

Increased glucose
production in liver

Hyperglycemia

Glucose
in urine

Excessive urination
Inadequate fluid intake

Dehydration

Severe hyperglycemia
(over 600 mg)

Lethargy
Mental Confusion
Shock

Hyperosmolar Hyperglycemic
Syndrome (HHS)

If Type 2 diabetes remains uncontrolled for a long period of time, more serious symptoms may result, including severe hyperglycemia (blood sugar over 600 mg), dehydration, lethargy, confusion, shock, and ultimately hyperosmolar hyperglycemic syndrome. This is more likely to occur in older people who have diabetes and in people suffering from an illness or infection. The main treatment is to replace lost fluids, which are usually given intravenously in the emergency room.

- Do not completely stop "forbidden" foods. Just limit the portions and times that you will eat that food.

- Don't shop for food when you are hungry.

- Exercise more. Choose several activities that you enjoy and plan to exercise at least four times a week.

- Keep the weight off by sticking to your new food and exercise plans. Don't go back to the old ones.

What Do I Do If I Get Sick?

Taking care of your Type 2 diabetes when you are sick can be difficult. Usually blood sugar increases when a person gets ill. If you cannot eat, it may be necessary to reduce or temporarily stop the amount of medication or oral hypoglycemic pills that you take (explained in Chapter 10). As always, the specific course of action to take when you are sick should be discussed with your healthcare provider.

Questions and Answers

Why Is It Important to Keep My Blood Sugar on Target?

With better control, you will have fewer complications.

If I Lose Weight, Will My Diabetes Go Away?

No. Diabetes cannot be cured, but it can be controlled, sometimes with diet and exercise alone. If you lose weight, your diabetes symptoms may disappear, but you will still have diabetes if your weight goes back up.

If I Take Oral Diabetes Pills, Do I Still Have to Follow a Meal Plan?

Yes. Even oral hypoglycemic pills cannot stimulate insulin production enough or reduce the need for insulin enough to make up for a careless diet.

Will I Have to Take Insulin by Injection?

There is no guarantee that your diet, or diet, exercise, and oral medications will always be able to control your diabetes; however, weight control and careful attention to diet and exercise increase your chances of staying in good control without having insulin injections.

What Should I Do If My Doctor Orders Laboratory Tests or Procedures That Require Me to Fast or Take Only Liquids or Clear Liquids Before the Test?

First, you will need to monitor your blood sugar more frequently to guard against hypoglycemia and hyperglycemia. Most often, you will need to stop taking oral agents (pills) for diabetes on the day that you start a liquid or a clear liquid diet. If your blood sugar is low, drink liquids with calories, such as apple juice or ginger ale. If your blood sugar is high, then drink sugar-free liquids. Take your diabetes pills as directed once your test is over, and plan to eat normal meals. People who take insulin are usually directed to take only half of their dose of insulin in the morning and afternoon or evening. Please ask your healthcare provider for directions that are specifically for you.

What Is My Target Blood Sugar?

Your target blood sugar should be individually determined. It is best to get your blood sugar closer to normal without getting frequent or significant low blood sugar (hypoglycemia). Other medical problems can interfere with your target blood sugar; thus, check with your healthcare provider for your blood sugar target.

For more information, check the American Diabetes Association's web site: http://store.diabetes.org, or call 1-800-232-6723.

CHAPTER 5

Monitoring

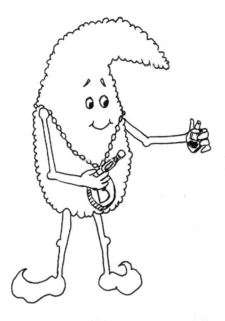

Self-Monitoring of Blood Glucose

Self-monitoring of blood glucose (SMBG) is a direct method of monitoring your blood sugar level and is your guide to diabetes control. At this time, all monitoring devices (except the Gluco-Watch) require a drop of blood (urine testing for sugar is an indirect method for measuring blood sugar that was used in the past but is seldom recommended today). You can test your blood sugar anywhere: at work, school, or home; on a plane, train, or a boat; or in your car. It's easy, fast, and quick.

SMBG is your guide to good control.

- An individualized target blood sugar range will be recommended.

- SMBG allows you to determine the pattern of blood glucose levels and to make necessary changes in your nutrition plan, exercise program, or insulin dose.

- With SMBG, you can measure the effects of changes in exercise, food, and insulin on your blood glucose level.

- SMBG helps you to avoid insulin reactions.

- The precise, immediate information that SMBG provides allows you to respond quickly to an elevation or decline in blood sugar.

- During an illness, the accurate information that SMBG provides can serve as a basis for treatment.

- Testing for ketones in your urine or blood also helps to determine insulin doses and treatment (explained later in this chapter).

When your healthcare provider recommends SMBG, he or she will prescribe a testing schedule (daily number of tests and times of day to test). You may be asked to test 1 to 4 times or up to 8 to 10 times a day. More tests are needed during illness or pregnancy or when intensive insulin therapy is used.

You may be asked to test at the following times:

When to test
Before meals
1-1/2 to 2 hours after a meal
At bedtime
At 3 a.m.
When you suspect a high or low blood sugar
Before and after exercise
Before driving and every 1 to 2 hours when driving long distances

- Before meals.
- One and a half to 2 hours after a meal.
- At bedtime.
- At 3 a.m.
- When you suspect a high or low blood sugar.
- Before and after exercise.
- Before driving and every 1 to 2 hours when driving long distances.

You may need fewer tests once you have established your blood glucose patterns. Remember, SMBG results are your guide to good control.

Equipment for SMBG

The following equipment is necessary for SMBG: a lancet device, lancets, test strips, a meter/sensor, alcohol wipes or soap and water, and a log book. A computer and software are optional for analyzing results that are stored in the memory of most meters.

SMBG Instructions

SMBG instructions vary depending on the meter that you use. Make sure that you carefully follow the instructions for your device. You first need to get a drop of blood (warm hands or a warm site makes a drop of blood easier to obtain). The side of the tip of a finger is the most frequently used site. Because using the same finger (or pair of fingers) causes calluses to build up, you'll feel less discomfort, but you'll need to be sure to obtain enough blood for each test. Some people prefer alternate testing sites (arms and thighs). This requires a cap change on the lancet device and a meter strip combination that is approved for alternate site testing.

These are the steps for obtaining a drop of your blood:

1. Follow the instructions included with your SMBG meter.

2. Wash your hands and the site with soap and warm water and dry completely, or clean the area with alcohol and dry completely.

3. Prick the chosen site with a spring-loaded lancet device and lancet.

4. If you are using your fingertip, hold your hand down, and milk the finger from the palm toward the tip. If only a small amount of blood appears, wait a couple of seconds and milk again. Do not squeeze close to the puncture. If using an alternate site, hold the lancet device tip against the skin until a small drop of blood appears.

5. Touch the drop of blood on the special test strip pad or designated area.

6. Record your test result.

What Should My Blood Glucose Levels Be?

Your personal goal depends on your age, the type of diabetes, how long you've had diabetes, other health conditions, lifestyle, and a desire for control. Here are some guidelines:

Time	Normal	Good Control	Needs Work
Before a meal (or fasting)	60 to 100 <110	90 to 130	Over 150 or under 70
Two hours after a meal	Under 140	Under 180	Over 200

These recommendations are from the American Diabetes Association; however, your healthcare provider will help you to set your own goals. For some people, a blood sugar level below 70 is too low, whereas for others, a level under

100 is too low. A level of over 120 before a meal is too high for some, whereas for others, it is acceptable. During pregnancy, the target is for the blood sugar range to be as close to normal as possible. Remember that you will not be able to achieve absolutely normal blood sugar all of the time. You will have some high and low blood sugars that will need to be corrected. Just don't give up working toward your target blood sugars!

Caution! An increase in the number of insulin reactions and the severity of insulin reactions may occur when tight control is your goal. For your safety, it is really important to monitor your blood sugar frequently and to work closely with your healthcare provider, as he or she will help you to identify patterns of blood sugar and to make adjustments in insulin, medications, activity, and food.

Caution! An increase in the number and severity of insulin reactions may occur when attempting tight control. Monitor your blood sugar frequently and work with your healthcare provider.

Recording SMBG Results

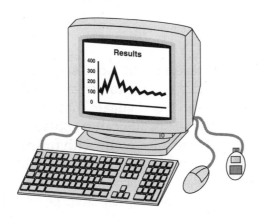

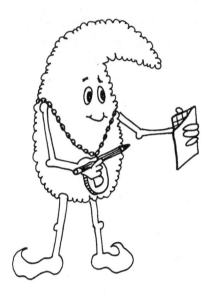

A record of your blood sugars or a computer-generated download from your meter is helpful. You and your health-care providers can use this information to make safe adjustments to your diet, exercise plan, and insulin or medication. Make sure that your SMBG test record includes any unusual events, such as illness, stress, and changes in exercise or activity level. For those working for tight control, you may be asked to keep more detailed records. This would include time, blood sugar, carbohydrate grams or food eaten, activity, and insulin.

SMBG Meters

Meters/sensors for testing your blood sugar level vary in the size, weight, test timing, range, and calibration method. They can read blood sugars that are as low as 0 and as high as 600 mg. Results can be obtained in 5 to 45 seconds. Up to 250 results, along with the date and time, can be stored in your meter. All of the available meters and sensors have been tested for accuracy. Costs vary from $50 to $100. Insurance coverage varies; thus, check with your insurance carrier. Trade-in offers and rebates can help to reduce costs. At this time, all meters require test strips, which cost about $0.65 each.

Photometric (color reflectance) meters have been around the longest and have proven reliable and accurate. They use a light source with filters and a lens to detect the color change on a strip. Glucose in the blood causes the color change. A digital result is produced.

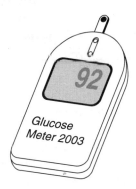

Another technology for glucose measurement uses electrochemical detection. Glucose in the blood causes a reaction on the test strip that produces a tiny current. The meter detects the current and reports a digital test result. Both types of meters have proven to be reliable and accurate.

Choosing a Meter

There are about 20 meters that are currently available. Constant improvements and updates are being made. Your healthcare provider can help you to select the best meter. Your vision, dexterity, need for quick timing, meter size, lighting, and ease of applying blood are assessed. One meter provides an extra feature for blood ketone testing. Lancet devices are provided with the meters. The replacement cost is $15 to $20.

The American Diabetes Association's *Diabetes Forecast* magazine publishes a yearly consumer issue and buyer's guide in which prices, accuracy, and comments about meters are available.

Ketone Monitoring

Testing for ketones is recommended for patients with Type 1 diabetes during illness and pregnancy and when blood sugars are uncontrolled. This test can be done on urine or blood. Test strips can be purchased at your local pharmacy. Your healthcare provider will show you how to test for ketones.

Why Should I Test for Ketones?

The presence of ketones is a warning that your body is using stores of fat to make fuel available to your cells. This occurs when insulin levels are too low or during starvation.

Glycosylated Hemoglobin A1c

Hemoglobin A1c is a test that reflects the average of your blood sugar levels over the past 2 to 3 months. It measures the amount of glycosylated hemoglobin, which is a protein that is found **inside of red blood cells.** Glucose (sugar) binds to hemoglobin, causing it to become **glycosylated.** The higher your average blood sugar was for the past 2 to 3 months, the longer the blood sugar remains elevated and the higher the percentage of glycosylated hemoglobin. The life of a red blood cell is about 3 months. You are constantly making new red blood cells as old ones die, and thus, your hemoglobin A1c level can change every 3 months.

Example A
Average Blood Sugar 90
HG B A 1 C 5.5%

H = hemoglobin
G = glucose

Example B
Average Blood Sugar 250
HG B A 1 C 8%

In these examples, the circles represent red blood cells; the large H inside the circles represents hemoglobin, and the small Gs represent glucose. Where a G is present in a cell, the hemoglobin is glycosylated.

The hemoglobin A1c tells your success in controlling blood sugar over the past 3 months, or it can be a reflection of all of the glycosylation that builds up, destroying nerves, eyes, kidneys, and blood vessels. A high hemoglobin A1c over a long period of time increases your risk of diabetic complications. A result near normal lets you know that you are controlling your diabetes, thus reducing your risk of complications. This test is done every 3 to 6 months, depending on your level of control and type of diabetes.

	Normal*	Goal	Needs Work
Hemoglobin A1c	4.6% to 6.0%	Less than 7.0%	More than 8.0%

*The normal value may vary depending on the method and the laboratory used.

Why Should This Test Be Done?

Knowing your average blood sugar can help you be motivated toward good control. It can also help you and your healthcare provider determine the effectiveness of your regimen over a long period of time. You and your healthcare provider will set your target goal. If you are not at your target for hemoglobin A1c, a change is needed.

If My Hemoglobin A1c Improves, Will the Complication Improve?

Some evidence shows that early complications may improve, but the more established complications will not get better; however, you can slow the progression of complications with improved control.

New Glucose Monitoring Systems

All people with diabetes will welcome the day when a device is available that constantly measures blood sugar and gives a number with the push of a button or just a glance. This will be a reality in the future. There are two systems currently available for continuous glucose monitoring. Both are intended for occasional, not everyday, use. They are also used to supplement, not replace, standard blood sugar testing.

The Medtronic MiniMed system consists of a monitor, cable, and sensor. The sensor is inserted just under the skin and taped into place. A cable connects the sensor to a monitor about the size of a pager. This monitor is worn for 72 hours. Up to 288 glucose values are measured each day and stored in the monitor. The results are downloaded in the clinic or physician's office. Graphs and charts display blood sugar trends and patterns. This information may help to guide your diabetes management.

The Gluco-Watch is also a continuous monitoring device. It looks like a large wrist watch and is worn on the forearm for a specified number of hours each day before the test pads need to be replaced. Every 20 minutes, an average blood sugar is displayed. This device is non-invasive (no needle puncture). Interstitial fluid glucose is drawn through the skin by a small current and is measured. Data from this device can also be downloaded and computer-generated charts printed to provide information that may help guide your diabetes management.

Research continues for new devices to monitor blood sugars and perhaps someday to signal an insulin pump to deliver just the right amount of insulin. The goal is to have both the pump and sensor implanted. These small devices are in human clinical trials at this time.

Questions and Answers

If My Blood Sugar Results Are Not Making Sense, What Should I Check?

Check for outdated test strips. Make sure to calibrate your meter to the test strips. Clean your meter periodically. Be sure you have an adequate blood sample. Do not expose test strips to heat and humidity. Do not leave the bottle of test strips open. Check that your meter and strips are using the brand-specific control solution.

What Are the Other Things My Healthcare Provider Will Monitor for Me?

- Microscopic amounts of protein in the urine that signal early kidney damage.

- Proteinuria, which are larger amounts of protein in the urine.

- Fructosamine, which is about a 6-week average blood sugar.

- Other blood tests to monitor your thyroid function, kidney function, and blood fats.

- Blood pressure.

Sample blood sugar logs are shown on the following pages.

Blood Sugar Log - Basic

Date	Breakfast	Lunch	Dinner	Bedtime	Notes:

Blood Sugar Log - Intensive Therapy

Date	Breakfast		Lunch		Dinner		Bedtime		Night	
	Before	After	Before	After	Before	After	Before	After	Before	After
Blood Sugar										
Insulin										
Carbs										

Date	Breakfast		Lunch		Dinner		Bedtime		Night	
	Before	After	Before	After	Before	After	Before	After	Before	After
Blood Sugar										
Insulin										
Carbs										

Date	Breakfast		Lunch		Dinner		Bedtime		Night	
	Before	After	Before	After	Before	After	Before	After	Before	After
Blood Sugar										
Insulin										
Carbs										

Date	Breakfast		Lunch		Dinner		Bedtime		Night	
	Before	After	Before	After	Before	After	Before	After	Before	After
Blood Sugar										
Insulin										
Carbs										

Date	Breakfast		Lunch		Dinner		Bedtime		Night	
	Before	After	Before	After	Before	After	Before	After	Before	After
Blood Sugar										
Insulin										
Carbs										

Date	Breakfast		Lunch		Dinner		Bedtime		Night	
	Before	After	Before	After	Before	After	Before	After	Before	After
Blood Sugar										
Insulin										
Carbs										

Date	Breakfast		Lunch		Dinner		Bedtime		Night	
	Before	After	Before	After	Before	After	Before	After	Before	After
Blood Sugar										
Insulin										
Carbs										

Blood Sugar Log - Pump Therapy

Date	Breakfast		Lunch		Dinner		Bedtime		Night	
	Before	After	Before	After	Before	After	Before	After	Before	After
Blood Sugar										
Carbs										
Bolus										
Basal Rate										

Date	Breakfast		Lunch		Dinner		Bedtime		Night	
	Before	After	Before	After	Before	After	Before	After	Before	After
Blood Sugar										
Carbs										
Bolus										
Basal Rate										

Date	Breakfast		Lunch		Dinner		Bedtime		Night	
	Before	After	Before	After	Before	After	Before	After	Before	After
Blood Sugar										
Carbs										
Bolus										
Basal Rate										

Date	Breakfast		Lunch		Dinner		Bedtime		Night	
	Before	After	Before	After	Before	After	Before	After	Before	After
Blood Sugar										
Carbs										
Bolus										
Basal Rate										

Date	Breakfast		Lunch		Dinner		Bedtime		Night	
	Before	After	Before	After	Before	After	Before	After	Before	After
Blood Sugar										
Carbs										
Bolus										
Basal Rate										

Notes: _____

_____

_____

CHAPTER 6

Nutrition

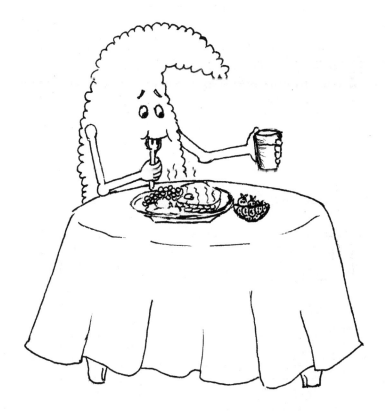

Healthy nutrition is the cornerstone of good diabetes care. Does this mean that you must follow a diabetic diet? No. The old "diabetic diet" has been replaced with well-balanced **meal plans** that are tailored to meet your individual needs, tastes, activity level, and lifestyle. Meal times, types, and amounts of foods are planned and adjusted for just you. You may need to learn more about foods, and you may have to make some changes in your eating habits; however, you won't have to give up your favorite foods. The better that you understand your meal plan, the more flexibility you can enjoy. Adults need enough calories to attain or maintain optimal weight. Children and adolescents need enough calories for growth and development. A growing teenager often requires many more calories than an adult. Children and teens receive a meal plan based on carbohydrate servings throughout the day. Your healthcare provider can help you to tailor favorite recipes to fit your meal plan and can teach you more about good nutrition and better health. Because your dietary needs are not like others, a dietitian is preferable because they have expertise. Once you understand your dietary needs, you'll be able to design your own menus and make good food choices.

Basic Nutrition

FOOD GROUPS	SUGAR CONVERSION
CARBOHYDRATES	100%
PROTEINS	60%
FATS	0%

Food contains many nutrients, including carbohydrates, proteins, and fats, which contain calories, as well as vitamins, minerals, and water, which contain no calories. Your meal plan will include all of the nutrients in amounts that promote good diabetes control, while providing adequate fuel for energy, and building and repairing your body.

Nutrients

Carbohydrate foods raise blood sugar the most quickly. When digested, carbohydrates turn 100% into glucose (sugar), which is the fuel your body burns for energy. There are two types of carbohydrate foods: simple and complex.

Simple carbohydrates include juice, fruit, honey, syrup, jam, candy, sugar, regular soda, desserts, and milk.

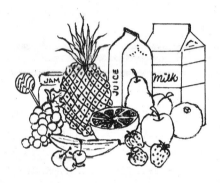

Complex carbohydrates include starchy foods such as pasta, rice, potatoes, cereals, breads, crackers, some vegetables, and dried legumes. These foods raise your blood sugar less if they are high in fiber.

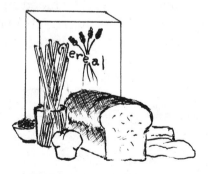

Protein foods build and repair muscle, organs, and body cells. They also provide fuel for energy. Protein, when digested, breaks down to amino acids. Approximately 60% of these amino acids get converted into glucose (sugar).

Protein comes from both animal and plant sources. Animal proteins include meat, fish, poultry, eggs, cheese, and milk. Plant sources include nuts, dried beans, legumes, and peanut butter. Protein is digested slowly and raises blood sugar about 3 to 4 hours after eating.

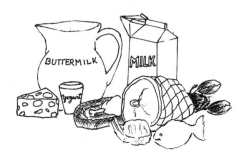

Fats in foods aid in the absorption of the fat-soluble vitamins: A, D, E, and K. When digested, fats are stored in fat cells and are later used as fuel for energy. They provide flavor and texture to food. Fat is high in calories, and excess fat increases the risk of obesity and heart disease. Fats are from animal and plant sources. Animal fat foods include butter, lard, bacon, cream, and the fat in meats, poultry, fish, eggs, and milk. Plant fats include cooking oils, avocados, nuts, and seeds. Fats are digested and absorbed the slowest (more than 8 hours) and have little effect on blood sugar, as only 10% or less is converted to blood sugar. Fats in foods slow the digestion and absorption of carbohydrate foods.

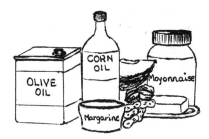

Some foods contain carbohydrates, proteins, and fats, including milk, yogurt, pizza, tacos, casseroles, and many prepared foods.

Calories

A calorie is a unit of heat that is used to express the energy-producing content of foods. Your dietitian will determine how many calories you need every day and how they should be divided among types of food, based on your height, weight, age, activity level, growth needs, metabolism, and general lifestyle. For example, an active young person of normal weight needs more calories than an inactive older person or an overweight person. Remember, if you eat more calories than you need to produce energy, the excess calories are stored as body fat.

Why Do I Need a Meal Plan?

If you have Type 2 diabetes, sticking to your meal plan helps you to achieve and maintain your weight goal and balances the foods that you eat with the insulin that your body produces, medications (or injected insulin), and exercise. If you have Type 1 diabetes, you will learn how to balance your meals and snacks with insulin injections and exercise and how to maintain a healthy weight.

Meal Planning

- Maintains blood sugar in your target range.
- Provides enough calories for optimal weight or growth.
- Helps to lower cholesterol as optimally as possible.
- May prevent or delay diabetic complications.

The purpose of meal planning is to provide a guideline of foods for healthy eating. There are many ways to create an individualized meal plan. When selected and designed especially for you, it will lead to good diabetes control and optimal weight.

Meal plans are generally based on one or more of the following methods:

- Carbohydrate counting.
- Exchange plan.
- Food pyramid.
- Plate method.

Your typical meal/snack plan may need only slight modifications, such as limiting the number of times that you eat out, using low-calorie snack foods, eliminating desserts, or controlling food portions. We do **not** recommend fad diets or diets that significantly restrict nutrients (e.g., a "protein-sparing diet").

Carbohydrate Counting

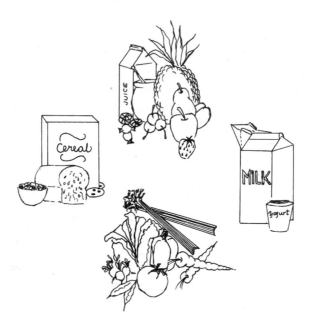

Carbohydrates have the greatest effect on blood sugar. Remember that 90% to 100% of carbohydrates turn into sugar, usually within 2 hours. This plan can be simple: counting carbohydrate choices or counting grams of carbohydrates (which is more complex). Some people eat consistent amounts of carbohydrates at each meal and snack, whereas others adjust premeal insulin to a more flexible plan. By monitoring your blood sugar, you will be able to learn your response to the carbohydrate counting meal plan. Your individualized plan is based on your blood sugar and weight goals, your exercise plan, your food preferences, and your desire for a more simple or flexible plan (for more information on carbohydrate counting, see the box on p. 94).

Exchange Plan

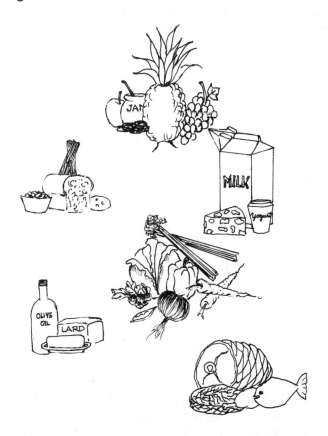

This method groups foods that contain similar nutrients. Exchange lists are groups of food that contain roughly the same mix of carbohydrates, proteins, fats, and calories.

Portions are weighed and measured to ensure specific serving sizes. This method provides a lot of structure and is the most useful for children, those working on weight reduction, or those who find structured diets helpful. The six exchange groups are starch, meat, vegetables, fruit, milk, and fat.

Sample 1,500-Calorie Diet	
Breakfast	**Afternoon Snack**
1 Fruit (List 4)	1 Fruit (List 4)
2 Starch/Bread (List 1)	**Dinner**
1 Fat (List 6)	2 Meat (List 2)
1 Milk (List 5)	2 Starch/Bread (List 1)
*Free Foods (List 7)	1 Vegetable (List 3)
Lunch	1 Fruit (List 4)
1 Meat (List 2)	2 Fat (List 6)
2 Starch/Bread (List 1)	*Free Foods (List 7)
1 Vegetable (List 3)	**Evening Snack**
1 Fruit (List 4)	1 Starch/Bread (List 1)
1 Fat (List 6)	1 Milk (List 5)
*Free Foods (List 7)	1 Fruit (List 4)

Food Pyramid

High-carbohydrate, low-fat diets promote higher blood sugar levels and increase the need for insulin. When monosaturated and polyunsaturated fats are added to the diet and refined carbohydrates are eliminated, the risk of heart disease is lowered.

The original food pyramid plan promotes a diet that is low in fat, sugar, and calories. Unfortunately, people who are following this diet tend to overeat foods that are in the starch group, especially the refined carbohydrates, such as white bread, rice, and pasta.

Researchers studied the effects of high-carbohydrate, low-fat diets and found that such diets promote higher blood sugar levels and increase the need for insulin. When monosaturated and polyunsaturated fats were added to the diet and refined carbohydrates were eliminated, the risk of heart disease was lowered. Based on these studies, two scientists from the Harvard School of Public Health developed a new food pyramid that promotes eating healthy fats along with whole grain foods. The refined carbohydrates, butter, and red meats are more limited.

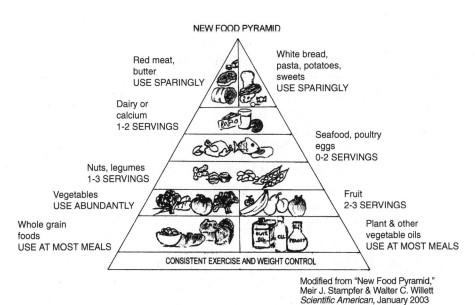

NEW FOOD PYRAMID

Red meat, butter
USE SPARINGLY

White bread, pasta, potatoes, sweets
USE SPARINGLY

Dairy or calcium
1-2 SERVINGS

Seafood, poultry eggs
0-2 SERVINGS

Nuts, legumes
1-3 SERVINGS

Vegetables
USE ABUNDANTLY

Fruit
2-3 SERVINGS

Whole grain foods
USE AT MOST MEALS

Plant & other vegetable oils
USE AT MOST MEALS

CONSISTENT EXERCISE AND WEIGHT CONTROL

Modified from "New Food Pyramid,"
Meir J. Stampfer & Walter C. Willett
Scientific American, January 2003

Plate Method

This plan is simple. You fill your plate with foods that are suggested in a diagram. It is basic and may be all you need.

Divide a 9-inch plate into fourths, then use moderate portions of suggested food groups in each of the four sections of the plate.

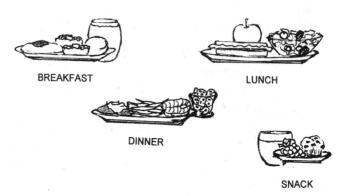

BREAKFAST

LUNCH

DINNER

SNACK

Reading Labels

You can select foods that are best suited for your meal plan when you learn how to read labels. Look for the information under "Nutrition Facts." First check the "Serving Size." Note the amount or size of the serving and also how many servings are in the package. The rest of the information is for the "amount per serving."

- Calories in each serving are listed first.

- Next, look for the **total carbohydrate** grams. The amount of carbohydrates from sugars may be listed under carbohydrates but are not counted separately. Multiply the total grams of carbohydrates by 4 to get the total calories from carbohydrates (15 grams of carbohydrates are in 1 slice of bread or in 1 medium fruit).

- Total fat grams are listed with the amount of saturated fat indicated. Less than 10% of your daily calories should come from saturated fat. Multiply the fat grams by 9 to get the total calories from fat.

- Total protein grams are also listed (7 grams of protein are in 1 ounce of meat). Multiply the grams of protein by 4 to get the total calories from protein.

Hearty Red Bean Stew

Nutrition Facts	
Serving Size 1 cup	
Servings Per Container About 3	

Amount Per Serving	
Calories 230	**Calories from Fat** 35
	% Daily Value
Total Fat 4g	6%
Saturated Fat 0.5g	3%
Cholesterol 0mg	0%
Sodium 680 mg	28%
Total Carbohydrate 38g	13%
Dietary Fiber 11G	44%
Sugars 9g	
Protein 11g	

Check with your dietitian or healthcare provider for individualized amounts that are recommended for you.

Obesity

If you are overweight, weight loss should be your primary goal. These methods help in weight loss: Eating fewer calories than your body needs for your usual activity level, and exercising because it helps to curb your appetite and burn calories.

One pound of fat is equal to 3,500 calories. To lose a pound in a week, you'd have to cut your calorie intake by 500 calories per day (500 calories × 7 days = 3,500 calories, or one pound). If that sounds like a lot of dieting for very little weight loss, remember that a pound a week is 52 pounds a year; however, you have to maintain these changes.

To achieve your ideal weight, you have to develop good eating habits; to maintain your weight, you must continue those habits. Be realistic. Making a big change in your life takes time. It might help to keep a record of your weight each week so that you know when you're making progress. Don't worry about occasional relapses. Don't be harsh with yourself if you overeat once or twice or regain a pound or two. Try to identify the causes of your relapses so that you can avoid them in the future.

Helpful Hints for Losing Weight

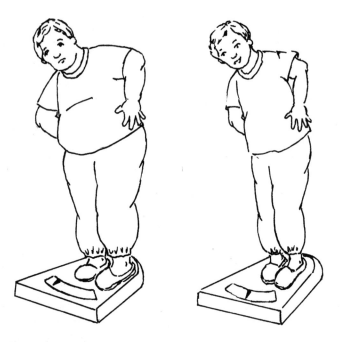

- Eat smaller meals more frequently throughout the day.

- Plan your meals so that you eat healthy food—not whatever is easiest.

- Think before you eat instead of raiding the refrigerator when you feel hungry.

- Use a smaller plate so that you won't take more than you want or need.

- Chew slowly and completely, savoring every mouthful.

General Guidelines

Eat Less Fat

- Cut down on red meat, and choose the leanest cuts. Eat more fish and poultry instead.

- Roast, bake, or broil instead of frying. Trim the fat off the meat and the skin off the poultry, and avoid adding fat when cooking. Beware of sauces and gravies because they often contain a lot of fat. Avoid fried foods.

- Eliminate or cut down on high-fat foods such as cold cuts, bacon, sausage, hot dogs, butter, margarine, salad dressings, lard, and shortening.

- Eat less ice cream, cheese, sour cream, cream, and other high-fat dairy products. Choose low-fat or lite versions (they're increasingly available in grocery stores). Drink skim or low-fat milk instead of whole milk.

Know Your Fats

Cholesterol is a fatty substance that is found in animal foods (meat, poultry, egg yolks, whole milk, cheese, ice cream, and butter). Have your cholesterol level tested; your goal is a level under 200 mg/dl.

High-density lipoprotein (good cholesterol) is a type of cholesterol that can protect against heart disease.

Low-density lipoprotein (bad cholesterol) is a harmful type of cholesterol that deposits on artery walls and increases the risk of heart disease.

Monounsaturated fat is a type of unsaturated fat that lowers blood cholesterol. It is found in olive and peanut oil.

Polyunsaturated fat is a vegetable fat that lowers total blood cholesterol. It is found in cottonseed, soybean, sunflower, and safflower oils.

Saturated fat is an animal fat that raises total blood cholesterol. It is found in hydrogenated vegetable fats, coconut and palm oils, cocoa butter, meat fat, whole milk, butter cream, and fatty cheeses.

Triglycerides are fats in the blood that may increase the risk of heart disease.

Increase Fiber

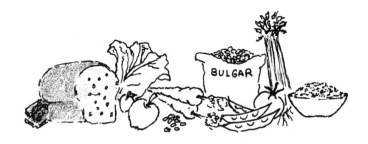

- Switch to whole-grain breads, cereals, and crackers.
- Eat more vegetables—both raw and cooked.
- Eat fresh fruit instead of juice.
- Include high-fiber foods, such as bran, barley, bulgur, brown and wild rice, and dried beans, peas, and lentils, in your diet.

Fiber Facts

Fiber is the part of plant foods that your body cannot digest.

Fiber relieves constipation, lowers blood cholesterol levels, and apparently slows the rate of carbohydrate digestion, reducing carbohydrate-induced elevations of blood sugar.

Fiber also causes gas if you eat too much too quickly; thus, add it gradually to your diet.

Limit Concentrated Sweets

- Avoid table sugar. Use an artificial sweetener that has no calories. Sweeteners without calories include saccharin (Sweet 'N Low), aspartame (Equal and Nutrasweet), sucratose (Splenda), and acesulfame-K (Sweet One).

- Limit honey, syrup, jam, jelly, candy, sweet rolls, regular gelatin, cake with icing, and pie. They contain a lot of calories in a small volume. Instead of fruit canned in syrup, choose fresh fruit or fruit that is canned in natural juice or water.

- Drink water or diet soft drinks. Regular soft drinks contain 8 teaspoons of sugar per can.

Other Food Facts

- Dietetic hard candy and diet chocolate contain about the same amount of calories as regular candy.

- "Diabetic foods" are not calorie free. They may have less sugar and sodium but more calories from fat.

- Fat-free foods are often higher in carbohydrates.

- Low-calorie foods usually contain 40 calories or less; low-fat foods contain 3 grams of fat or less.

Alcoholic Drinks

Discuss the use of alcohol with your healthcare provider. For most people with diabetes, alcohol can be safely used if your diabetes is in control; however, alcohol is high in calories and has no nutritional value, stimulates appetite, may interfere or change the action of some medications, can be harmful to a fetus, may cause low blood sugar, is digested as a fat and may raise high-density lipoprotein cholesterol, and can worsen nerve disease (neuropathy).

Tips for Safe Use of Alcohol

- Use only in moderation and sip slowly.
- Drink only with meals or snacks.
- Never eliminate a meal to balance alcohol calories.
- Avoid sweet mixed drinks and sweet wines.
- Do not drink before or after exercise.

Alcoholic Beverages and Calories

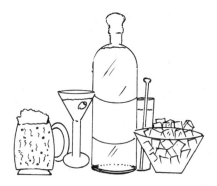

Beverage	Serving Size	Approximate Calories
Beer, 4.5% alcohol	12 ounces	110
Dry wine	4 ounces	70
Lite beer	12 ounces	90
Gin, rum, scotch, vodka, whisky	1.5 ounces	80 proof = 96, 100 proof = 120

Eating Out

Eating at a restaurant or at a friend's home is enjoyable. You can still go out to eat and stay in good control if you remember a few tips:

- Know your meal plan—especially carbohydrate portions. Estimate portions as best you can.

- You don't have to finish everything on your plate. Take some home.

- Food often has hidden fats. Beware of sauces, gravies, and casserole-type foods.

- Try to order plainly cooked foods (baked, steamed, or broiled).

- Look for "heart-healthy meals" on the menu.

- Share a dessert.

- If the meal is delayed, eat a **small carbohydrate** snack such as crackers, bread sticks, or juice.

Fast Food Restaurants

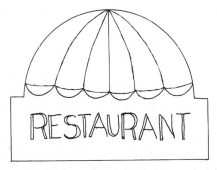

Fast foods are generally inexpensive and very high in saturated fats, calories, and sodium. A double cheeseburger, fries, and a milk shake can quickly put you over the top of your total calories and carbohydrates for the day. A small hamburger, a diet drink, and a salad with low-calorie dressing would be a better choice. If you do splurge, make it infrequent. Many pocket guidebooks are available that give specific information on the carbohydrate, protein, and fat content of foods on the menu at fast food restaurants. Fast food restaurants have nutrient composition of their menu choices on their web sites, and the nutrient composition is also available on posters and brochures in the restaurants. More fast food restaurants are now offering low-fat choices to their customers. Thus, think before you order.

Tips for Feeding Children with Diabetes

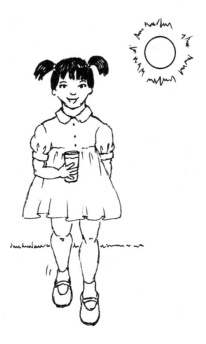

- Dilute fruit juices for greater volume, especially in the summer.

- Sometimes children won't eat a certain food. Eventually, the phase will pass if it doesn't become a battle. Continue to offer small portions of a variety of foods.

- For the nonmilk drinker, try flavored yogurts, cottage cheese, or puddings.

Changing Eating Behavior

Here are some tips to help you manage the way you eat.

- Make changes gradually. Don't try to do everything at once. It may take longer to accomplish your goals, but the changes you make will be permanent.

- Set realistic, short-term goals. If weight loss is your goal, try to lose 2 pounds in 2 weeks, not 20 pounds in 1. Walk two blocks—not two miles—in the beginning. Success will come more easily, and you'll feel good about yourself!

- Reward yourself. When you achieve a short-term goal, treat yourself to a movie, buy a new shirt, read a good book, or visit a friend.

Resources: Available at the American Diabetes Association Bookstore

The Common Sense Guide to Weight Loss. Barbara Caleen Hansen, PhD, and Shauna S. Roberts, PhD.

Diabetes Meal Planning Made Easy. Hope Warshaw, MMSc, RD, CDE.

Sweet Kids. How to Balance Diabetes Control and Good Nutrition with Family Peace.

Month of Meals: *Classic Cooking*
                    Old Time Favorites
                    Meals in Minutes
                    Vegetarian Pleasures
                    Ethnic Delights

Snack, Munch, Nibble, Nosh Book. Ruth Glick.

ADA Guide to Healthy Restaurant Eating. Hope Warshaw, MMSc, RD, CDE.

Carbohydrate Counting for Persons with Diabetes (video). Available at American Diabetes Association Bookstore: 1-800-232-6733.

Carbohydrate Counting: Getting Started (Level 1), Moving On (Level 2), Using Carbohydrate/Insulin Ratios (Level 3). Booklets available at the American Diabetes Association Bookstore: 1-800-232-6733.

The Diabetes Carbohydrate and Fat Gram Guide. Lea Ann Holzmeister, RD, CDE.

Cooking with the Diabetic Chef. Chris Smith.

How to Use Carbohydrate Counting: What Foods Do I Count?

- Foods that are high in carbohydrates are in the starch, fruit, and milk groups. Vegetables are low in carbohydrates and do not need to be counted unless you eat more than 1.5 cups.

- Each carbohydrate choice is about 15 grams. Although counting carbohydrate choices is not as accurate as counting grams, this may be adequate for you. Discuss the best method with your dietitian or healthcare provider.

Sample List			
Food	1 Choice (15 grams)	2 Choices (30 grams)	3 Choices (45 grams)
Bread	1 slice	2 slices	3 slices
Cereal, plain	1/2 cup	1 1/2 cups	2 1/2 cups
Pasta and sauce	1/2 cup	1 cup	1 1/2 cups
Potatoes	1 medium or 1/2 cup	1 large or 1 cup	1 extra large or 1 1/2 cups
Rice	1/2 cup	1 cup	1 1/2 cups
Juice	1/2 cup	1 cup	1 1/2 cups
Peach	1 medium	1 large	1 extra large
Milk	1 cup	2 cups	
Ice cream	1/2 cup	1/2 cup	1/2 cup (high fat)
Yogurt	1 cup plain	1 cup with fruit	1 1/2 cups with fruit
Cookies			
Oreos	2	4	6
Lorna Doones	2	4	6
Chips Ahoy	2	4	6
Cake	1 small piece, no icing	1 medium piece, no icing	1 medium piece with icing
Pie	1/8 single-crust pie	1/8 double-crust pie	1/6 double-crust pie
Granola Bar	1/2	1	1 1/2
Brownie	Unfrosted 2" square	Unfrosted	Frosted

You will need a list of carbohydrate foods from your dietitian or healthcare provider and can also purchase a carbohydrate-counting booklet at any bookstore.

Read the label on packages for the amount of carbohydrate grams per serving. Divide the number of grams by 15 to get the number of carbohydrate choices.

Example: Carbohydrate per serving = 60 grams
60 divided by 15 = 4 choices (you may need to round off this number)

Example 1: Breakfast

1	English muffin	30	
1 Slice	Cheese	0	
1	Black coffee	0	
1/2 cup	Juice	15	(45 ÷ 15 = 3)
		45 grams or 3 choices	

Example 2: Lunch

1	Juice popsicle	15	
1	Tuna sandwich	30	
Handful	Pretzels	15	
	Diet soda	0	(60 ÷ 15 = 4)
		60 grams or 4 choices	

Example 3: Dinner

1	Cup mashed potatoes	30	
1	Roll	15	
5 oz	Chicken	0	
1 1/2 cup	Green beans	15	
8 oz	2% Milk	12	
1	Medium apple	15	(82 ÷ 15 = 5.4)
		82 grams or 5 1/2 choices	

We recommend a visit with your dietitian for an individualized carbohydrate counting plan and for a comprehensive list of foods.

Carbohydrate Counting for People Who Are on Intensive Insulin Therapy

Another way to use carbohydrate counting is to equate insulin with grams of carbohydrates. An insulin-to-carbohydrate ratio is used. This approach allows for the most flexibility in choosing the amount of carbohydrates that you want to eat at each meal and/or snack. Fast-acting insulin is taken before each meal or snack. Checking a blood sugar 1.5 to 2 hours after the meal will indicate if the dose is correct. Most people need one unit of fast-acting insulin for every 10 to 15 grams of carbohydrates. However, this may vary from 1 unit per 5 to 20 grams. Your ratio may also be different for breakfast, lunch, and dinner.

Insulin-to-carbohydrate ratios must be individualized. To determine your insulin-to-carbohydrate ratio, add your usual total daily dose of insulin, and divide this number into 450.

Example 1: Total daily dose is 30 units $450 \div 30 = 15$
The insulin-to-carbohydrate ratio is 1 unit for 15 grams of carbohydrates.

Example 2: Total basal insulin   22 units
Average of daily bolus doses   + 23 units
Total daily dose   = 45 units
$450 \div 45 = 10$ The insulin-to-carbohydrate ratio is 1 unit for 10 grams of carbohydrates.

Remember, these are only guidelines to begin. Monitoring your blood sugar provides the information for adjusting ratios. This method takes time and effort but has great rewards. Remember that the amount of fat and fiber in foods can affect blood sugar. You may also have success following a Weight Watchers Program or another commercial plan; although one of these plans is likely good, check with your healthcare provider before beginning.

CHAPTER 7

Exercise and Activity

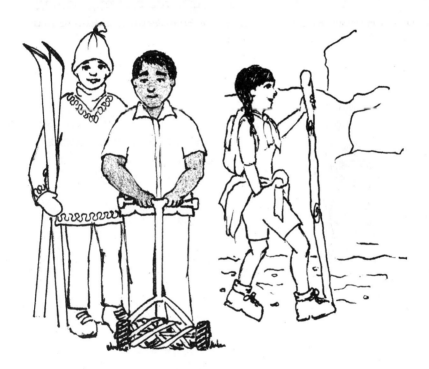

Regular physical activity is recommended for everyone, but for people with diabetes, it is one of the cornerstones of good diabetes care. Check with your healthcare provider before starting an exercise program, as he or she will want to check for any problems that require a modification in your exercise program (e.g., you may need a stress test or orthotics). Remember, start any program slowly and gradually build up the time and intensity.

 Exercise is one of the cornerstones of good diabetes care.

Types of Exercise and Activities

There are three forms of exercise: aerobic, strengthening or anaerobic, and stretching. A well-rounded exercise program includes all three forms.

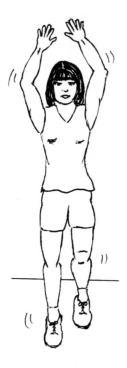

- Aerobic exercises work the larger muscles and increase heart rate and respirations (your heart beats fast and you breathe harder).

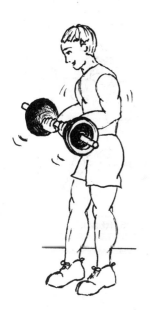

- Strengthening/anaerobic exercises work muscles against resistance. Weight machines, free weights, and calisthenics are used.

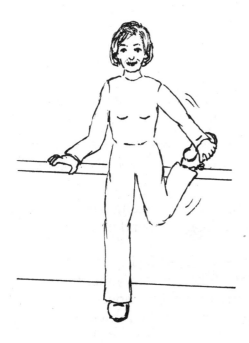

- Stretching muscles improves flexi-bility.

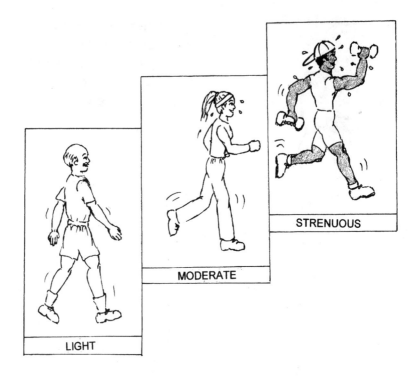

STRENUOUS

MODERATE

LIGHT

Levels of Exercise

- Light exercise, such as slow walking, will increase your heart rate but not your breathing.

- Moderate exercise, such as tennis, will increase both your heart rate and breathing. You'll know you're getting a workout.

- Strenuous exercise, such as running a long race, will substantially increase your heart rate and breathing.

Some activities are not generally classified as an exercise but may involve some or all of the previously mentioned forms of exercise. These activities include household chores or yard work or some types of jobs. Activities burn calories as well as give your body exercise and should not be overlooked when trying to maintain blood sugar control.

Types of Aerobic Exercise			
Exercise	Example of Activity	Intensity	Benefits
Aerobic	Walking Jogging Biking Roller blading	Increases with energy output and length of time	Lowers blood pressure, improves stamina/endurance
Strength	Free weights Weight machines Interval training	Increases with weight being moved or amount of resistance	Improves overall exercise performance and strength
Flexibility	Stretching/ Yoga	Low intensity	Iproves range of motion and balance

Exercise is best when done four to seven times a week for 20- to 60-minute sessions. Keeping your blood sugar in control during and after exercise will take some planning and practice.

Effects of Exercise

- Improved blood sugar control.

- Less need for diabetes medication.

- Reduced body fat.

- Reduced stress.

- Possible prevention of Type 2 diabetes.

- A decreased risk of cardiovascular disease.

Do not exercise when you have any of these problems:

- Blood sugar that is under 100 mg (take additional carbo-hydrates first).

- Blood sugar that is over 300 mg with urine ketones (urgent need for insulin).
- Illness.
- An active retinopathy (or have had recent laser surgery).

Keep Safe

- Drink adequate fluids.
- Wear proper socks and shoes.
- Carry a medical identification.

Selecting an Exercise Program and Activities

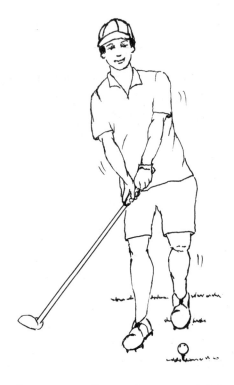

First, decide what types of exercise or activities you like. What have you enjoyed in the past? Do you have a friend with whom to exercise? Is there a gym or a track nearby? Can you join any clubs that focus on exercise? You may want to select several types of exercise or activities and vary them according to the season, weather, or time required. Don't pick walking on a treadmill if it bores you because you'll end up making excuses not to do it. If you love music and dancing, you may want to sign up for dance lessons. No partner? Try line dancing. If you dislike any form of exercise but love being outside and gardening, this could work for you. Select something and get started!

Tips to Get Started

- Be realistic—you can't run before you walk.

- Go slowly—you may need to start with only 10 minutes a day.

- Plan your exercise/activity time on your calendar or day planner.

- Track your progress.

- Plan the frequency—how often you will exercise or engage in the activity each week; the duration—how long you will do it; and the level of intensity—light, moderate, or strenuous.

- Consult with an exercise physiologist if possible.

How Many Calories Can I Burn in an Exercise Session?

The number of calories burned during exercise depends on your size and on the type, duration, and intensity of your exercise. Light-intensity exercise for 30 minutes burns 100 to 120 calories and includes casual walking, light housework, dancing, yoga, swimming, and golf. Moderate-intensity exercise for 30 minutes burns 150 to 200 calories and includes cycling at 10 miles per hour, gardening, vacuuming, washing floors, bowling, canoeing/kayaking, horseback riding, volleyball, low-impact aerobics, walking at 5 miles per hour, square dancing, and ice skating.

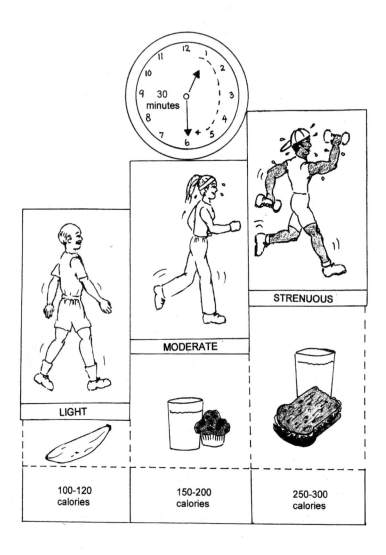

Strenuous exercise for 30 minutes burns 250 to 300 calories and includes jogging at 5 miles per hour, roller blading, downhill skiing, mountain hiking, squash/handball, cross-country skiing, tennis singles, chopping wood, and shoveling.

Prevent Hypoglycemia

If you take insulin, carry glucose tablets or try a sports drink that has been half diluted with water.

Tips for Aerobic Exercises

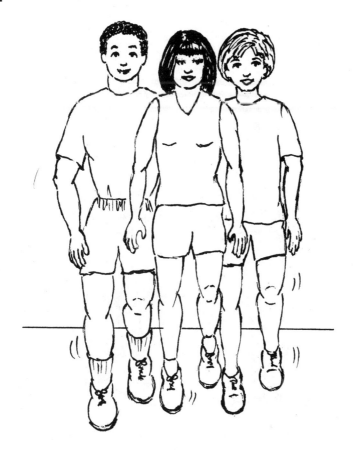

- Don't exceed your target heart rate.
- Slow down if you cannot talk.
- Set your own pace if you are in a group. You don't need to keep up with anyone else.
- Warm up and cool down for 10 minutes each.

- Wear good, supportive shoes.
- Wear double socks or cushioned socks that wick away moisture.
- Wear proper exercise clothes to wick away moisture.
- Wear suggested protective gear.

Tips for Strengthening Exercises

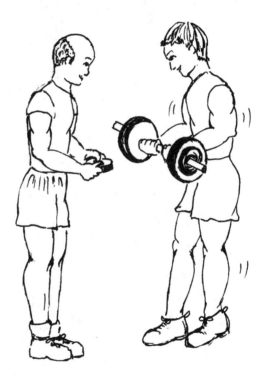

- Learn the right technique.
- Work with a partner if lifting weights.
- Exercise two to three times per week for 20 to 30 minutes each session.
- Allow at least 1 day of rest between doing the same exercise.

Tips for Stretching

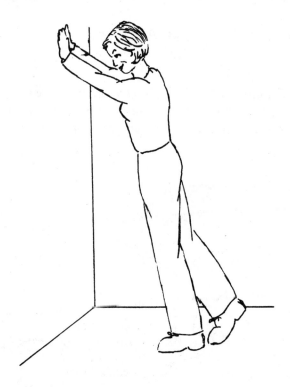

- Warm up and cool down by doing 5 to 10 minutes of mild aerobic exercise.

- Stretch only as far as you can without pain.

- Hold the position for 8 to 10 seconds.

- Do not bounce.

- Breath in and out slowly.

- Use smooth, flowing motions.

Additional Exercise Information

Options to Increase Activity

 Walking is an ideal exercise no matter your age. It's safe, inexpensive, and requires less strength than many sports, and you don't need lessons!

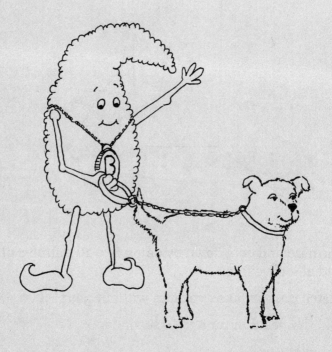

Many practical ways to increase your activity are available. Walking is one of the easiest: You can walk to the store instead of driving, walk the dog, park farther from your destination and walk the rest of the way, and get off the bus a stop or two early and walk the extra few blocks. Walking is an ideal exercise no matter your age. It's safe and inexpensive and requires less strength than many sports, and you don't need lessons to begin. You can walk alone or with others, indoors or outside.

For safe walks, wear appropriate shoes that have plenty of support. Never go barefoot. Wear loose-fitting clothing and dress in layers that you can remove if you get hot. Start slowly and increase your distance and pace each week. Take long, easy strides and breath deeply. Carry some fast-acting sugar and be aware of low blood sugar symptoms. In hot weather, bring extra fluids. Always check your feet for injuries after walking.

In addition to walking, there are other ways of being active that don't even seem like exercise. Take the stairs instead of the elevator. When watching television, get up and move around during commercials. Use hand-opcrated (rather than electric) appliances. Mow the lawn, rake the leaves, or wash the car—even washing windows or floors can provide good exercise and can burn calories.

Easy Exercises for Beginners

Bending and stretching exercises are good for beginners because they are easier and are less likely to cause injury than more strenuous aerobic exercises. Even after you advance to more strenuous activities, it's a good idea to prepare for each workout with a few minutes of stretching. To avoid injury, always do 5 minutes of a warm-up exercise, such as light walking, before your stretch. In addition to stretching, there are safe beginner's exercises that you can do lying down on your bed or a floor mat or sitting in a chair. When stretching, stand with your legs apart and bend forward, backward, and to each side. These are some exercises that you can do lying down on your bed or a floor mat:

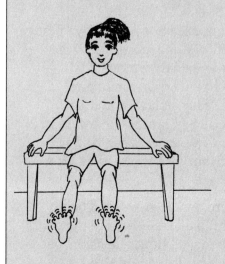

- Wiggle and circle toes of both feet.

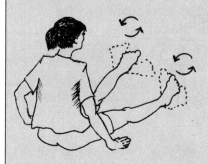

- Circle each foot, first in one direction and then in the other.

- Do knee raises by lying on your back. Bring one knee up as close to your chest as possible and then lower it slowly. Repeat with the other knee.

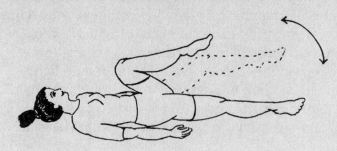

- While lying on your back, raise your arms as high over your head as you can. Stretch and then slowly roll side to side.

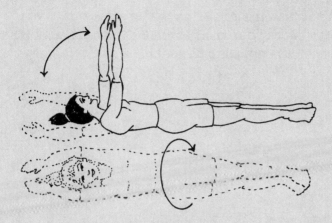

- While lying on your back, take a deep breath. As you exhale, lift your head and shoulders.

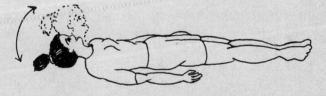

- While lying on your side, raise one leg and move it in a circular pattern. Turn and repeat with the other leg.

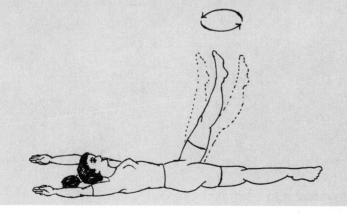

These exercises can be done while sitting in a chair:

- Raise both arms in front of you. Make a big circle with each arm, first in one direction and then in the opposite direction. Next, stretch your arms out to your sides. Move your arms in circles in one direction and then in the opposite direction.

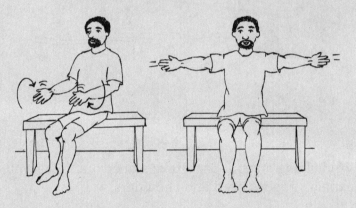

- While seated, push down on the arms of your chair and try to lift your body off the seat.

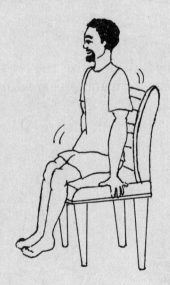

- Try armchair exercise videos.

Exercise for the Overweight Person with Type 2 Diabetes

You may not feel like exercising because you are tired and because moving takes a lot of effort; however, you'll feel better when your diabetes is in good control, and you can help make this happen by following your diet and by exercising. Exercise decreases your appetite and helps your own insulin to work better. Exercise also burns up food calories and calories that are stored in your body as fat. By burning more calories than you eat, you'll lose weight, and when you lose weight, you'll be able to move with less effort.

Monitoring Blood Sugar During Exercise

When beginning an exercise program, check your blood sugar before, during, and after exercising (see Chapter 5). By monitoring your blood sugar, you can do these things:

- Learn your body's response to exercise.
- Avoid hypoglycemia.
- Determine an appropriate pre-exercise snack.
- Carry glucose.

Exercise Chart

Date	Exercise	Duration	Intensity	Before BS	After BS

For People Who Take Insulin

Balancing Exercise with Food or a Decrease in Insulin

People who take insulin injections will need to adjust insulin and/or add snacks. Discuss your options with your healthcare provider. The longer and harder that you exercise, the more carbohydrates you will need for energy. Even with extra snacks, some people will need to decrease insulin also. By monitoring your blood sugar closely, you will quickly learn what works for you.

Guidelines for Balancing Exercise/Activity with Snacks (Must Be Individualized)

(For every 30 minutes)

Intensity	Blood Sugar	Snacks	CHO
Low	Under 100	1 fruit or one-half cup of juice	15 g
	More than 100	Nothing	0 g
You may need 10 g of carbohydrates (1/2 cup of juice) for an additional 30 minutes.			
Moderate	Under 100	2 pieces of fruit or 1 cup of juice	30 g
	100 to 200	1 fruit or one-half cup of juice	15 g
	More than 200	Nothing	0 g
Add 10 to 15 grams of carbohydrates (one-half cup of juice) every additional 30 minutes.			
Strenuous	Under 100	1 cereal bar and 1 cup of juice	45 g
	100 to 200	1 cup of juice or cereal bar	30 g
	More than 200	One-half cup of juice	15 g
Add 30 g of carbohydrates (1 cup of juice or sports drink) for every additional 30-minute period. For long duration exercise, you will need to add protein and fat.			

Check the carbohydrate content in sports drinks, cereal bars, and power bars. They are handy snacks.

Safety Tips

- Keep well hydrated. Drink water before, during, and after exercise.
- Check feet for any redness, cuts, blisters, or bruises before and after exercising.
- Do not exercise if your blood sugar is over 300 mg and you have ketones.
- Do not exercise when ill.
- Stop exercising immediately if you get light headed, dizzy, nauseated, or weak, or have chest pressure, pain, leg cramps, indigestion, loss of coordination, or uneven heartbeat.
- Listen to your body. Stop for a brief rest when necessary.
- Check blood sugars frequently.
- Adjust insulin according to a plan discussed with your healthcare provider.

For People on Pump Therapy

You have the best method for adjusting insulin for planned and spontaneous exercise. For light exercise and activity of short duration, no change is usually necessary. For long durations, or more intensity, you may need to decrease both basal rates and bolus doses by 20% to 50%.

Team Sports

It is nearly impossible to predict the amount of calories a person will burn in various team sports, as there are too many variables. How long will he or she play? Will the person sit out most of the game? For these situations, it's best to have lots of quick snacks, sports drinks, bars, and glucose tablets available for minute-to-minute changes. Checking blood sugars frequently will give you information on how well you are balancing your blood sugar with exercise.

Why Do Insulin Reactions Sometimes Occur Hours After Exercising?

During periods of strenuous exercise, your body consumes substantial amounts of muscle and liver glycogen. It can take some time to replace this glycogen; during this time, your blood glucose level may drop.

If your blood glucose is high after strenuous exercising, avoid taking extra insulin right away. During the cool down or recover phase, the blood sugar will frequently fall on its own. Check blood sugars frequently. Extra insulin may cause a severe insulin reaction hours later. Obtaining blood sugars after exercise is the best insurance against this.

What Exercises Should I Avoid If I Have Diabetic Complications?

If you have significant diabetic complications, you may be advised to avoid heavy lifting, high-impact aerobics, or strenuous, long-duration exercise. A better choice would be moderate walking (for those without foot problems), stationary biking, cardioglide equipment, and armchair exercise videos. We advise you to check with your healthcare provider. You don't want to do damage to your body. The benefits mentioned earlier can still be of value to you, but you'll need to go more slowly and less intensely. Remember to check your blood sugars frequently.

Can I Exercise If I'm Pregnant?

Don't start a strenuous program once you are pregnant. If you have been exercising before pregnancy, you will want to limit the strenuous part of your workout to less than 15 minutes.

- Check with your healthcare provider and obstetrician before beginning a new program.
- Drink lots of water.
- Monitor your blood sugar frequently.
- Keep your heart rate under 140 beats per minute.
- Contractions may indicate that you are working too hard.
- Focus on breathing.
- Avoid high-impact exercises.
- Lying on your back may cause a quick drop in blood pressure.
- Avoid sudden stops and starts and twisting.
- Try walking, swimming, yoga, Tai Chi, or mild stretching exercises.

How Can I Exercise If I Travel a Lot?

Try to stay at motels and hotels with exercise facilities or a pool. Ask about safe areas to walk and jog. If you camp, you're in an ideal situation for evening walks and treks.

Does Child's Play Count as Exercise?

Yes! Biking, roller blading, skateboarding, and swimming are just a few fun activities for kids. Encourage sports of all kinds. Limit TV and computer games. Classes for gymnastics, dance, or martial arts are great for children.

Resources

Diabetes Exercise and Sports Association
P.O. Box 1935
Litchfield Park, AZ 85340
1-623-535-4593
1-800-898-4322
http://www.diabetes-exercise.org/

Books

The Diabetic Athlete. Sheri Colberg.

Handbook of Exercise in Diabetics. Neil Ruderman, MD, John Devlin, MD, and Stephen Schneider, MD.

The Diabetic's Sports and Exercise Book. June Biermann and Barbara Toohey.

CHAPTER 8

Insulin

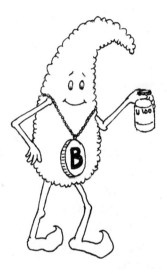

If you have Type 1 diabetes, your body produces no insulin, and you must thus receive insulin by injection. If you have Type 2 diabetes, you may need insulin injections if your diabetes cannot be controlled with meal planning, exercise, and oral medication. Remember that insulin cannot be taken orally because it is protein that would be broken down during digestion.

Insulin is measured in units. A unit is a measure of weight: 100 units = 3.6 mg. There are 100 units of insulin in 1 cc of solution (called U100 insulin). There are 1,000 units in a bottle of U100 insulin. U100 insulin is used with U100 insulin syringes. In rare instances, U500 may be needed. Some people may need to dilute their insulin to half strength or U50.

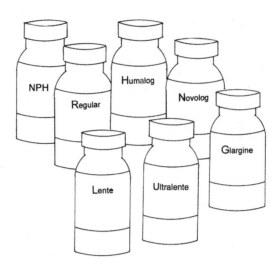

Types of Insulin

Human insulin has now replaced all previously used animal insulins. Human insulin is genetically engineered from nonpathogenic E. *coli* bacteria or yeast buds. Three companies make insulin: Eli Lilly makes Humulin N, L, and R and Humalog. Novo Nordisk makes Novolin N, R, and Novolog. Aventis makes Lantus (insulin glargine). Insulins are characterized by their **action.**

Action	Names of Insulin
Rapid/short acting	Lispro (Humalog); Aspart (Novolog); Regular (Humulin R and Novolin R)
Intermediate acting	NPH (Humulin N and Novolin N); Lente (Humulin L and Novolin L)
Long acting	Ultralente (Humulin U); Glargine (Lantus)
Combination of intermediate and rapid or short acting	Humulin 70/30; Humalog mix 75/25; Novolin 70/30; Novolog mix 75/25

The important characteristics of each type of insulin are as follows:

- When it starts to work (**onset**).

- When it works the hardest (**peak activity**).

- How long it lasts (**duration**).

Factors such as the injection site and the exercise level affect the onset, peak, and duration of insulin. **Lispro and Aspart insulin** have the fastest onset and the shortest duration. It is taken before meals and snacks to lower a high blood sugar quickly. Insulin pumps use only fast- and rapid-acting insulins. **Regular insulin** is fast acting and lasts a short time in the body. It is used before meals to control the after-meal rise in blood sugar and to lower blood sugar quickly when an immediate correction is needed. **NPH insulin** contains added protamine for an intermediate-acting effect. NPH insulin provides a basal amount of insulin. Two (sometimes three) injections a day are usually prescribed. **Lente insulin** contains added zinc, which gives it an intermediate-acting effect that is similar to NPH. Lente insulin also provides a basal amount of insulin. Two injections a day are usually prescribed. **Ultralente insulin** contains a lot of added zinc to give it a longer-acting effect. Ultralente insulin provides basal amounts of insulin. One to two injections a day are used in combination with Humalog, Novolog, or regular insulin before meals. **70/30 Insulin** is a mix of 70% NPH and 30% regular insulin. Two injections a day are usually recommended. **75/25 Insulin** is a mix of 75% NPH and 25% Humalog or Novolog. It is used two to three times a day before meals. **50/50 Insulin** is a mix of 50% NPH and 50% regular insulin. Two or three injections are used before meals. **Insulin glargine** is basal, long-acting insulin with no peak action. It is taken only once a day. Lantus (glargine) is **never** mixed with other insulins in the same syringe. Often fast-acting insulin is injected before each meal.

Insulin Activity			
Type	Onset	Peaks	Duration
Aspart (Novolog)	≈15 minutes	30–90 minutes	Less than 4 hours
Lispro (Humalog)	5–15 minutes	45–90 minutes	Less than 5 hours
Regular	30–60 minutes	2–4 hours	4–6 hours
NPH (N)	1–1.5 hours	4–10 hours	14–18 hours
Lente (L)	1–2 hours	6–12 hours	16–20 hours
Ultralente (U)	4–6 hours	12–16 hours	20–24 hours
Insulin glargine	1–2 hours	None	24 hours+
70/30 Mix	30 minutes	2–3 hours and 8–12 hours	18–24 hours
50/50 Mix	30 minutes	2–3 hours and 8–12 hours	14–18 hours
75/25 Mix	5–15 minutes	1 hour and 6–10 hours	14–18 hours

ACTIVITIES OF INSULIN

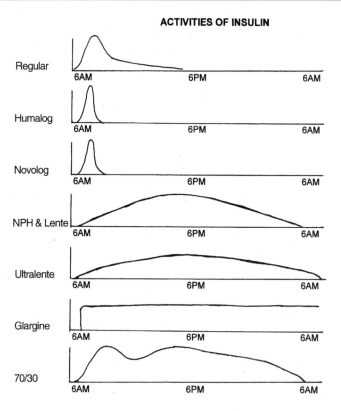

Many combinations of insulin may be used
to balance your meals and activity level.

Your Injection Schedule

Follow the schedule of insulin injections that your health-care provider prescribed because it is precisely matched to your activity and meal plan. You may also be given a scale to increase your Humalog, Novolog, or regular insulin when your blood sugar is high.

Your Insulin Doses

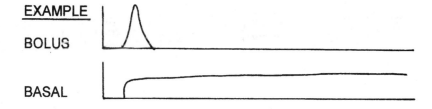

The types and amounts of insulin recommended for you will try to provide an insulin profile that is similar to how you once made insulin. Before you had diabetes, your beta cells made a steady amount of insulin throughout the day. This is called basal insulin. Each time that you ate a meal or snack, your beta cells would produce a burst of insulin so that you could use the food for energy. This is called the bolus dose. If you still make some insulin, you may need only intermediate- or long-acting insulin once or twice a day. If you make absolutely no insulin, you may need intermediate- or long-acting insulin plus three or four fast- or short-acting insulin injections before meals each day.

	FOOD	Increases Blood Sugar ⬆
	INSULIN	Decreases Blood Sugar ⬇

Many ways are possible to combine and mix insulins. Your insulin doses will also be based on your insulin sensitivity, your exercise/activities, and your food intake. You will need to monitor your blood sugars, record your test results, and discuss with your healthcare provider any changes that are needed to meet your target blood sugar levels.

Storing Insulin

 Always have extra insulin on hand. Fast-acting insulin should be kept for emergencies and sick days, as well as syringes, needles, and alcohol wipes.

You may keep opened bottles of insulin at room temperature for 1 month (less than 86°F). Insulin loses potency when exposed to temperature extremes; thus, don't leave it on a sunny windowsill or in the freezer. Store unopened bottles in the refrigerator, and rotate your supply so that you use the oldest bottles first.

Always have an extra bottle of insulin on hand. Keep rapid- or fast-acting insulin on hand for emergencies and sick days, even if you do not inject it daily. Also, keep a good supply of syringes, needles, and alcohol wipes.

- Before injecting insulin, always check the expiration date on the bottle. Do not use insulin after the expiration date.

- If insulin is exposed to freezing temperatures or to temperatures above 85°F or 30°C, throw it away.

- If insulin contains small, hard, white particles that do not mix or that look stringy, throw it away.

- If insulin sticks to the bottle, creating a frosted appearance, throw it away.

Injecting Insulin

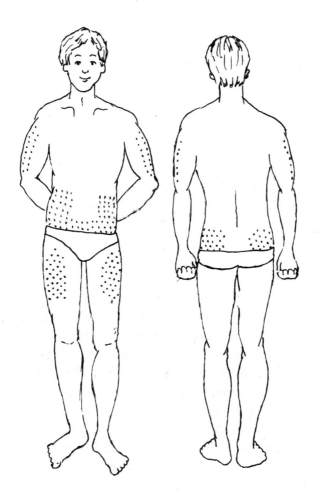

Injection sites include the abdomen, outer upper arms, thighs, buttocks, or hip areas. Do not inject insulin near bony places or joints or give injections closer than 1 inch apart. Insulin absorption can vary from site to site. The best absorption site is the abdomen. Exercise may alter the absorption of insulin from the arms, legs, and buttocks. Do not inject near an exercised muscle. Select a site for each time of the day that you will be injecting. Rotate the injections 1 inch apart within that site.

Preparing for Injection

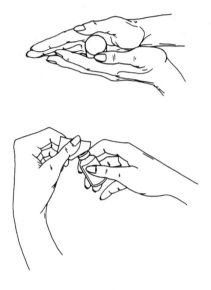

Steps for preparing your syringe differ depending on whether you use one type of insulin or a mixture of two or more insulins. Intermediate- and long-acting insulin—except Lente—should be rolled first, as in the picture above. Always clean the top of the insulin bottle with alcohol before you insert the needle. If you use just one type of insulin, draw up air into the syringe that is equal to the amount of your dose. Insert the needle through the rubber stop and push air into the bottle. Invert and draw back the plunger to your insulin dose.

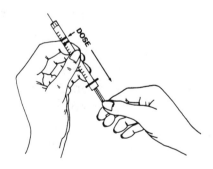

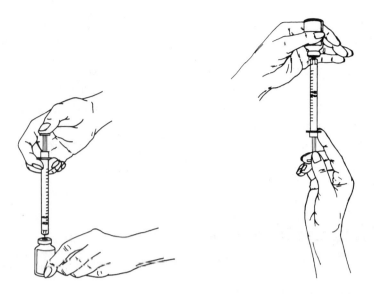

Tap the syringe to raise any air bubbles to the top. Push the plunger up and draw again to the proper dose.

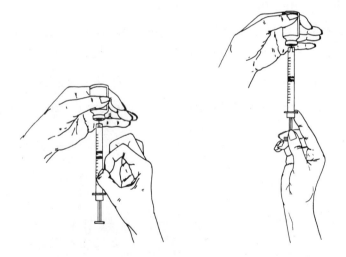

If you use more than one type of insulin, draw up air equal to the dose of intermediate- or long-acting, cloudy insulin. Push the needle through the rubber stop and push the plunger down. Take out the needle empty. Now draw up air equal to the amount of fast-acting regular, Humalog, or Novolog. Push the needle into the rubber top of the clear insulin and push the plunger down. Now invert and draw the plunger back to the correct dose.

Tap the syringe to raise any bubbles to the top. Push some insulin back into the bottle and draw back again to the correct dose of fast-acting insulin (clear). Remove the needle and carefully reinsert the needle into the cloudy insulin and add the dose of N, L, or U to the fast-acting regular, Humalog, or Novolog. **Never mix Lantus (glargine) with any other insulin.**

Giving the Injection

- Select the site.
- Clean the site with alcohol.
- Pinch up your skin between your thumb and forefinger.
- Hold the needle close to your skin.
- Insert the full length of the needle with a quick motion.
- Push the plunger completely down.
- Release the pinched skin and remove the needle.
- If insulin tends to leak out, hold pressure on the site for 3 seconds.

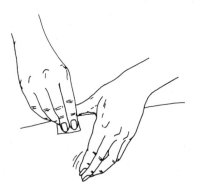 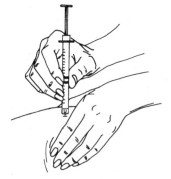

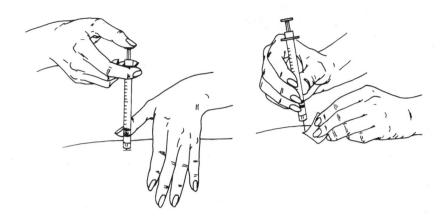

Reactions to Injected Insulin

Occasionally you may notice at the injection site a small, hard, red area that may also itch. This is a mild allergic reaction that will go away in a day or so. A more generalized allergy to insulin causes hives and itchy skin over other parts of the body. This is very rare and usually disappears by itself. If the itching continues, consult your healthcare provider.

- **Insulin edema** (swelling) may develop when you start insulin therapy. You may notice swelling in your legs, ankles, feet, hands, or face. It is usually not severe and will go away in a few weeks.

- **Lipohypertrophy** is the formation of scar tissue in an area that has been used repeatedly for injection. A firm, lumpy area develops. Insulin absorption is changed in this area. This condition is seen less frequently with the use of human insulins.

- **Lipoatrophy** describes the "pitted" areas that may form at injection sites. This condition, now rare, resulted from loss of fat in the area due to repeated injections with impure insulins.

Syringes and Needles

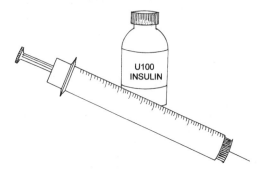

Use needles and syringes once and then discard. A variety of syringe/needle sizes exists. Several companies make syringes. Your insurance company may cover only one brand.

Syringe Size	Holds	Needle Sizes	Needle Length
3/10 cc	30 units	30 G, 31 G	5/8-inch traditional 3/8-inch short
1/2 cc	50 units	29 G, 30 G	5/8-inch traditional 3/8-inch short
1 cc	100 units	29 G, 30 G	5/8-inch traditional 3/8-inch short

When writing a prescription for your insulin needles, your healthcare provider considers the following:

- Your insulin dose (the syringe size needs to be appropriate for holding your dose of insulin).

- Your ease in reading the unit scale (small amounts are easier to read with 3/10 cc).

- Your dexterity (ease of holding the syringe—larger syringes may be easier to hold).

- Whether you are thin or heavy (the short needles are great for children or thin adults but are not good for obese people).

Injection Aids

Magnifiers are available at most pharmacies for those who have difficulty reading the unit scale. Spring-loaded injectors will quickly stick the needle in—you still need to push the plunger. Jet injectors are needle-free devices that inject pressurized insulin through the skin without a needle. They are expensive and are usually not covered by insurance. They can cause bruises in thin people and can take more time to learn to use. Devices are also available for people who are legally blind. A social worker or the Commission for the Blind in your area can help to locate a certified instructor.

Insulin Pens and Injection Devices

Insulin pens look like a heavy-duty writing pen. There are also a number of new devices of all shapes and sizes that hold a cartridge of insulin and allow you to dial up a dose of insulin. Some are disposable, whereas others use an insulin cartridge. Insulin pens/cartridges hold 150 U or 300 U of insulin. A disposable needle is screwed to the tip of the cartridge before injection. Pens and devices are user friendly, convenient, easy to carry, and assure dose accuracy. The needles come in the traditional length of 1/2 inch or the short length of 1/3 inch.

Disposing of Syringes, Needles, and Lancets

Check with your city or county for any specific laws and directions. If none are in effect, dispose of syringes, needles, and lancets in a puncture-proof container, such as an empty laundry liquid detergent bottle or bleach bottle with a screw-on cap. Some people use coffee cans, but the tops need to be taped on before disposing into the trash. Used syringes, needles, and lancets are considered medical waste. Do not toss them into a trash bag. The improper disposal of syringes and needles is illegal and hazardous.

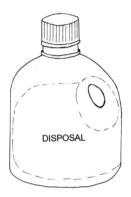

 Dispose of used syringes, needles, and lancets according to local laws regarding medical waste disposal. If there are no laws in effect, use a puncture-proof container, such as an empty laundry liquid detergent bottle or bleach bottle with a screw-on cap.

Insulin Reactions: Hypoglycemia

An insulin reaction is an unpleasant side effect of insulin that occurs when diet, exercise, and insulin are out of balance. Normal blood sugar levels are between 60 and 110 mg/dl. When you have an insulin reaction, your blood sugar may fall below 60 mg/dl, may fall rapidly from a higher to a lower level, or may simply fall below your usual level. This is called **low blood sugar** or **hypoglycemia** (hypo = too little, glyc = sugar, emia = blood). An insulin reaction can occur if you do the following:

- Inject or bolus too much insulin.

- Skip a meal, eat too little, or wait too long between meals.

- Exercise or work more than usual without adjusting insulin or food.

Symptoms of an Insulin Reaction

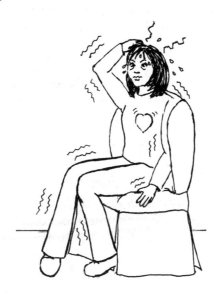

When you have an insulin reaction, the symptoms come on suddenly.

Stage	Signs and Symptoms	Response
Mild	• Pale, cold sweat and clammy feeling • Dizziness, weakness, or shakiness • Hunger • Pounding heart or rapid heart rate	Hormone response
Moderate	• Irritability, impatience, anger • Personality change • Nervousness or confusion • Blurred or double vision • Decreased mental ability • Slurred speech	Brain dysfunction
Severe	• Convulsions/loss of consciousness (not common)	

An insulin reaction is your body's response to low blood sugar. When your brain senses low blood sugar, it signals the release of hormones called catecholamines. One such "catecholamine" is adrenaline! Catecholamines produce the effects of pallor, sweating, shaking, a pounding heartbeat, nervousness, and irritability. Catecholamines also cause the release of stores of sugar in the liver (glycogen), which raises your blood sugar.

Neuroglycopenia

Your brain needs glucose to function. As blood sugar drops, many of the brain functions are altered. This alters your usual brain function, causing you to become confused, irritable, unreasonable, and eventually, if not treated, unconscious.

Treating an Insulin Reaction Yourself

Do not wait to see whether symptoms will go away.

- Take some kind of **fast sugar food** to raise your blood sugar quickly. Treat **before** testing your blood sugar.

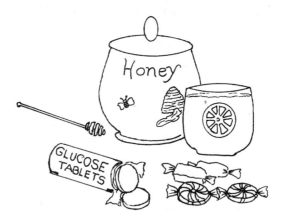

- Stop what you are doing and sit or lie down.

- Wait 15 minutes. If you do not feel better, treat and test your blood sugar again.

Do not overtreat a reaction by continuing to eat until symptoms go away or by eating anything in sight. You need only a small amount of fast-acting sugar to correct the problem.

These are some of the fast sugar foods that are easy to find:

From the Drug Store (These Work the Fastest)
Insta-Glucose (1 tube)
Glutose (1 tube)
Glucose tablets (3 to 4)
Dex Tabs (3 to 4) (come in flavors)
Monoject Insulin Reaction Gel (1 packet)

From the Grocery Store (These Take More Time to Work)
Life-Saver candies (4 to 6)
Cola or other soda (6 ounces)
Honey or corn syrup (2 tablespoons)
Fruit juice (4 ounces)
Jelly beans (6 to 10)
Sugar (2 teaspoons or 2 packets)

Always carry a fast-acting sugar with you. After a reaction, you may feel tired, have a bad headache, and have high blood sugar. **Do not make a permanent change in your insulin dose at this time. Try to identify the cause of the reaction.** If you have frequent insulin reactions at the same time of day, you may need to increase food intake or lower insulin amounts. Keeping a record of blood sugar tests, insulin doses, exercises/activity, insulin reactions, and how you feel will help you and your healthcare provider make adjustments.

Preventing Insulin Reactions

- Remember to balance your food, exercise, and insulin.
- Test blood sugars more frequently when your usual schedule varies or when exercising.
- If your meal is delayed, eat a small snack.

Hypoglycemia Unawareness

Hypoglycemia unawareness is the inability to detect low blood sugars. No symptoms of sweating, shaking, or an increased heart rate warn the person that his or her blood sugar is getting dangerously low. Catecholamine hormones don't kick in to warn of a low blood sugar. The first symptom may be mild confusion, a lack of coordination, behavior changes, fatigue, or sleepiness. If you have hypoglycemia unawareness, others may note that you look pale and "glassy-eyed" or that you are acting strangely.

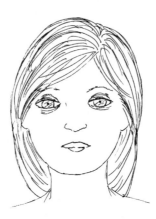

Who Is More at Risk for Hypoglycemia Unawareness?

- People who have had diabetes for more than 10 to 15 years.
- People who are on intensive insulin therapy with tightly controlled blood sugars.

- Those who experience frequent low blood sugars (especially during pregnancy).

- Those on certain medications that block normal reactions (e.g., beta blockers).

Can This Be Corrected?

 Learn to recognize hypoglycemia. Light-headedness, fatigue, hunger, or difficulty thinking can be warning signs. By being more aware, you may be able to detect your personal warning symptoms.

It may be possible to restore some mild awareness by training people to be more "tuned in" to early warning signs. Another way is to target higher blood sugars for 3 to 4 weeks and then slowly tighten control. If you have hypoglycemia unawareness, the following tips will help you:

- Test your blood sugar frequently during the day.

- If you awaken for any reason during the night, test.

- Always test before driving.

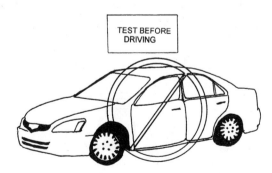

TEST BEFORE DRIVING

- Tell those with whom you associate about the warning signs and how to help.

- Teach family or a close friend how to give you glucagon if needed (discussed later in this chapter).

- Learn your first signal of falling blood sugar.

- Treat before testing, even with a vague symptom.

- Practice operant conditioning—this is training that makes you automatically respond to a body signal. For example, are you getting irritable? If so, reach for glucose tablets.

You may be able to increase your awareness of hypoglycemia: Anytime your blood sugar is 70 or below, stop and think about how you are feeling. Do you notice any light-headedness, fatigue, hunger, or difficulty thinking? Focus on any vague symptoms that you have. When you feel this happen again, treat and then test. By being more aware, you may be able to detect your personal warning symptoms.

More Information on Hypoglycemia

Teach your family, friends, teachers, and coworkers how to spot and help with a reaction. If you ignore reaction warning symptoms and do not take sugar, you could become unconscious. Although this is unlikely, you can protect yourself by teaching family and friends how to give a glucagon injection in an emergency (the instructions are given below).

Glucagon Injection Kit (Solution in Syringe)

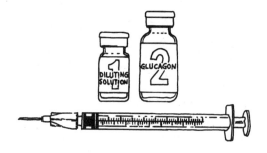

1. Inject all of the solution into an ampule.

2. Shake to mix.

3. Draw into the syringe.

4. Inject into the upper arm, thigh, or buttocks.

Tips on Assisting a Person Who Is Experiencing Hypoglycemia

Do not directly confront the person. Remember that a person who is having an insulin reaction may be agitated and hostile. Often someone experiencing a reaction may also be unable to recognize the symptoms and may get angry if you mention that he or she is having a reaction. Try a gentler tactic. Approach from the side. You may try saying, "Let's stop for something to drink," or "would you like to join me for a juice break?" Try to learn what works best for that person. You might even ask him or her what would be most helpful to say and do. Be sure to ask when the person is **not** having a reaction! Never force fluids or foods if the person is unconscious or **unable to swallow.** Give glucagon if it is available and you've been instructed in technique. If glucagon is not available, rush the unconscious person to the hospital or call 911.

Questions and Answers

How Serious Is Hypoglycemia?

You can easily treat hypoglycemia (insulin reaction) with fast-acting sugar. Even before you take sugar, your body begins to correct the sugar imbalance. The catecholamines (mentioned previously here) that are released during a hypoglycemia episode cause the liver to release stored glycogen, which converts to glucose and raises your blood sugar. Only prolonged, severe hypoglycemia (less than 20 mg for over 1/2 hour) can result in damage to the brain or the heart. This is very rare.

What Is a Somogyi/Rebound Effect?

A Somogyi/rebound effect occurs when your liver releases a lot of stored glycogen in response to a reaction; high blood sugar results. This creates an overcorrection. High blood sugars that respond poorly to insulin, urine ketones, and a feeling of exhaustion for a day after a reaction indicate a Somogyi/rebound effect.

How Can I Tell If I Have Slept Through a Nighttime Insulin Reaction?

You will awake with a high blood sugar and a headache and will feel exhausted. You may have had bizarre nightmares, night sweats, and restless, poor sleep.

Adjusting Insulin Doses

Life is always changing. People gain weight, lose weight, start a new exercise program, change jobs, have children, and endure illnesses and other stresses. All of these things will alter your insulin doses. You can learn how to spot the need for adjustment and how to adjust your insulin doses.

The three basic causes of blood sugar fluctuation are diet, insulin, and exercise; however, there are a multitude of reasons:

- Insulin error.
- Changes in weight.
- Some medications.
- Changes in exercise or activity level.
- Food added, omitted, or delayed.
- Illness or infection.
- Alcohol consumption.
- Insulin injected into a lumpy area or an exercising arm or leg.

- Overtreatment of an insulin reaction.

- Skipped insulin injection or loss of insulin potency.

Two types of insulin adjustments include permanent adjustments based on blood sugar *patterns* and temporary adjustments to correct a high blood sugar. Permanent insulin adjustments are based on blood sugar patterns. A pattern occurs when your blood sugar is in the same range at the same time of the day for 3 consecutive days. This could be on target or above or below target.

Blood Glucose Level				
Day	Morning	Noon	Afternoon	Bedtime
Monday	179 mg	136 mg	97 mg	147 mg
Tuesday	166 mg	129 mg	84 mg	141 mg
Wednesday	209 mg	145 mg	92 mg	159 mg

Although the numbers are different each day, you can see a pattern. Morning blood sugars are all over 140, and afternoon blood sugars are all under 100. In this case, an increase in the evening NPH, Lente, Ultralente, or glargine insulin will lower your blood glucose in the morning. When your blood glucose level fluctuates, try to identify the cause of the high or low blood glucose result.

Pattern Management

Your diabetes educator can help you learn how to adjust your own insulin doses according to high and low blood sugar patterns. Here are the steps:

1. Once you have observed a pattern of high or low blood sugars at the same time on 3 successive days, determine what insulin should be working at that time. Consult the insulin summary chart that is presented earlier in this chapter for information on insulin peak times and durations.

2. Adjust your dose of that insulin by 10% of your total daily dose (some people may need a 20% dose adjustment): Increase insulin for high blood sugar, and decrease insulin for low blood sugar.

3. Change only one type of insulin at a time.

4. Check the effect of your insulin adjustment for 3 days before making another adjustment.

5. Children may require only 0.5-unit changes.

6. Adjust insulin only if your healthcare provider has given you the "go ahead."

This diagram summarizes the steps:

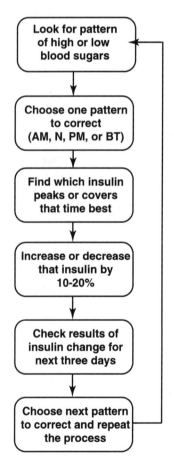

Pattern of High Blood Sugars

Date	AM	Noon	PM	BT
			201	
			252	
			220	

Pattern of Low Blood Sugars

Date	AM	Noon	PM	BT
	52			
	48			
	59			

Time Blood Sugar Out of Range	Adjust This Insulin
Before breakfast	Evening intermediate- or long-acting
Before lunch	Morning fast/rapid-acting
Before dinner	Morning intermediate- or long-acting or lunch fast/rapid-acting
Bed time	Before dinner fast/rapid-acting
3 a.m.	Bedtime intermediate- or long-acting or before dinner long-acting

A pattern may also be corrected by a change in your meal plan or exercise program. Talk with your healthcare provider for help in making adjustments of insulin and food.

Temporary Correction of a High Blood Sugar

High blood sugars that occur sporadically (no pattern) can be corrected with additional fast/rapid-acting insulin. You will need to use one of these three methods to determine your correction dose:

1. The insulin scale.

2. An insulin-to-blood sugar ratio based on "the 1,500 rule."

3. The 10% to 20% dosing method.

The insulin scale is used before meals (not at bedtime) and is based on a blood sugar result. The insulin amount increases as the blood sugar goes up. The insulin scale may look like this. Your healthcare provider will fill in the doses of fast/rapid-acting insulin:

Insulin Scale Chart			
Blood Sugar	Breakfast	Lunch	Dinner
Under 100			
101–150			
151–200			
201–250			
251–300			
301–350			
351–400			
Over 400*			

If you are **not** eating a meal, you will need another scale:

Blood Sugar	Insulin (fast/rapid)
Under 100	
101–150	
151–200	
201–250	
251–300	
301–350	
351–400	
Over 400*	

*Call your healthcare provider if your blood sugars are not responding to extra insulin or if blood sugars remain over 400 mg.

The 1,500 Rule (+1800 Rule) is a system that was developed by a diabetes doctor to estimate the drop in blood sugar that occurs with each unit of regular or Humalog insulin. This is also called the "Insulin Sensitivity Factor."

To calculate your sensitivity factor:

1. Add up your total daily dose of insulin.
2. Divide 1,500 by the total daily dose: total daily dose ÷ 1,500.
3. The result is the "sensitivity factor."

This provides a ratio of insulin to blood sugar.

1. Add up all of your usual insulin doses.

   Example:

Breakfast	16 units U
	8 units H
Lunch	6 units H
Supper	12 units U
	8 units H
	50 units total daily dose

2. Divide 1,500 by the total daily dose of 50:

$$\frac{30}{50)\overline{1500}} = \text{insulin sensitivity factor}$$

3. The result is the **sensitivity factor.**

This means that 1 unit of Humalog will lower the blood sugar by 30 mg.

Write down the target blood sugar (e.g., 100). This is the number you want your blood sugar to be.

Now, let's put it together:

Example

Actual blood sugar	190
Minus target	−100
Result	90

Divide the result by the insulin sensitivity factor of 30:

$$\frac{3 \text{ units}}{30 \overline{)\ 90}} = \text{correction dose}$$

In this example, 3 units would lower the blood sugar to the target of 100.

Now, let's try your numbers:

Total daily dose _____ divided into 1,500.

You insulin sensitivity factor is _____.

Next, your blood sugar _____

Minus your target blood sugar = _____

Amount that needs correction _____

Amount that needs correction ÷ insulin sensitivity factor = units of extra insulin

Percentage Dosing

Percentage dosing also uses a person's total daily dose of insulin as the basis. Ten percent of the total daily dose is used to correct a high blood sugar; 20% of the total daily dose is used to correct a high blood sugar *plus* ketones.

Example

1. Insulin Program

Breakfast	12 units N
	4 units R
Lunch	0
Dinner	6 units R
Bedtime	8 units N
	30 units total daily dose

2. 10% of 30 units is 3 units

   20% of 30 units is 6 units

Use 10% for blood sugars over 150 and 20% for blood sugars over 250 plus ketones.

Fill in your numbers:

Total daily dose = _____

10% _____ Use for blood sugar over 150

20% _____ Use for blood sugar over 250 plus ketones

Try to identify the cause of the high blood sugar. Check the "Causes of High and Low Blood Sugar" chart.

Intensive Insulin Therapy

(You may skip this part if you are not using or interested in intensive insulin therapy.)

Intensive insulin therapy is designed to imitate the normal release of insulin from the beta cells. It attempts to keep blood sugar levels as close to normal as possible. Regular, Humalog, or Novolog insulin is injected before each meal to match the rise in blood sugar from carbohydrates eaten. This is called a **bolus dose**. N, L, U, or glargine (Lantus) is injected once or twice a day to provide a steady amount of insulin. This is called the **basal dose**(s). Insulin pump therapy is the most effective method of delivering basal and bolus doses of insulin (p. 151).

What Is Involved?

- Diabetes self-management.
- Three or more insulin injections a day or insulin pump therapy.
- A meal plan based on carbohydrate intake or insulin calculated to cover the amount of carbohydrates selected for the meal or snack (see Chapter 6).
- Bolus dose insulin that is adjusted for exercise/activity.

- Monitoring blood sugar before each meal, at bedtime, before and after exercise, and occasionally 1.5 to 2.0 hours after meals and at 2:00 to 3:00 a.m.

- Striving to achieve your personalized blood sugar targets and hemoglobin A1c targets through blood glucose data analysis.

- Correcting blood sugars four or more times a day.

- Typically, target blood sugars are under 100 before meals, are less than 140 at 2 hours after meals, and are greater than 100 at 3:00 a.m.

- Flexibility for meals, snacks, and exercise/activity.

What You Will Need to Do

- Learn how to count carbohydrates (see Chapter 6).

- Determine your insulin-to-carbohydrate ratio.

- Determine your insulin sensitivity factor (discussed previously in this chapter).

- Learn your blood sugar response to exercise/activity.

- Explore insulin pump therapy.

Once you are educated, you can begin. You will calculate and give your bolus doses (fast/rapid-acting insulin) and evaluate the effectiveness of your basal insulin (intermediate- or long-acting insulin). Long-acting insulin is given once a day with rapid-acting insulin given before each meal.

Why Choose Intensive Insulin Therapy?

- Empowerment in that you will be in charge of your diabetes control.

- Greater flexibility in eating, exercising, and working schedules.

- A greater sense of well-being and satisfaction.

- A better rapid response to out-of-target blood sugar.

Insulin Pump Therapy (Continuous Subcutaneous Insulin Infusion)

Do you have unpredictable blood sugars even if you follow the same day-to-day schedule and meals? Do you experience low blood sugars without warning, for no apparent reason? Is your hemoglobin A1c higher than you or your healthcare professional would like? Are you tied to your diabetes schedule of meals and injections? Have you just given up trying because, no matter what you do, your diabetes remains uncontrolled? There are thousands of people just like you. Over 200,000 people with diabetes have solved these problems by changing to insulin pump therapy. They revel in the freedom and flexibility that pump therapy allows while benefiting from improved glucose control.

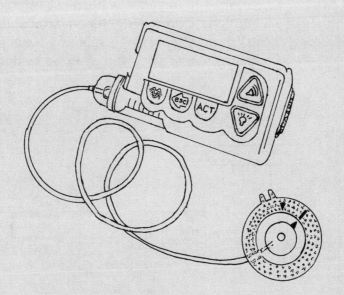

What Is an Insulin Pump?

The insulin pump is a small battery-operated device that uses computer chip technology to deliver insulin continuously (basal) and when activated in a burst (bolus). A compartment holds an insulin reservoir that is connected to an infusion set. At the end of the infusion set, a fine-gauge needle is used to insert a flexible canula; the needle is then removed. The canula is taped in place and is used for 48 to 72 hours. The pump is worn 24 hours a day. Some people prefer to remove it temporarily when bathing, during contact sports, and for other special circumstances. Pumps are approximately 2 × 3 inches or smaller. Only fast/rapid-acting insulin (Humalog, Novolog, or Velosulin) is used in the pump. The object of pump therapy is to mimic the action of normal beta cells by delivering preprogrammed basal rate profiles and delivery of activated bolus doses.

Basal insulin allows for background insulin to be delivered continuously between meals and during the night. Basal insulin can be programmed to increase or decrease at predetermined times to accommodate for dawn phenomenon and to prevent hypoglycemia during the night. Temporary basal rates may also be set for changes in activity and exercise, or during illness.

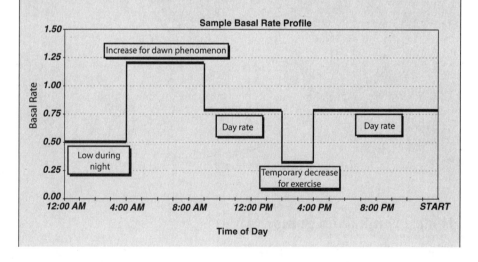

Bolus doses are activated to cover the rise in blood sugar after meals or snacks, or when more insulin is needed to correct a high blood sugar. The bolus dose can be increased or decreased to match the food you choose. Bolus doses can be delivered immediately (normal), spread out over a selected time of 1 to 8 hours (square), or divided, with part of the dose given immediately and part of the dose spread out over several hours (dual). Bolus doses are calculated based on insulin-to-carbohydrate ratios and on insulin sensitivity factors. New software in some pumps will do the calculations for you.

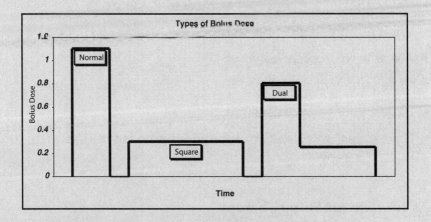

Will I Still Have to Test My Blood Sugar?

Yes. The insulin pump is an "open loop system," meaning there is no feedback to the pump to tell it what to deliver. No glucose sensor is in the pump. People using pump therapy must test their blood sugar a minimum of four times per day. One must calculate bolus doses based on carbohydrate ratios and a sensitivity factor. Basal rates are individually determined and are based on blood sugar patterns. Soon, blood glucose meters will be able to beam the test result directly to the pump so that the pump can calculate the correct dose.

Will Pumps Ever Be Implanted?

Yes. In the future, both the pump and the glucose sensors will be implanted. This will be a "closed loop system" where the sensor provides the feedback on blood sugar to the pump. Research is being conducted now to make this a reality.

The ideal candidates for pump therapy

- Are highly motivated.
- Are responsible and reliable.
- Have a desire for improved control of diabetes.
- Want a more flexible lifestyle.
- Are able to problem solve.
- Have sufficient dexterity.
- Have a good support system.
- Have access to a healthcare provider who is familiar with pump therapy.

Advantages of Pump Therapy

- Improved Hgb A1c.
- Improved sense of well-being, lifestyle, and flexibility.
- Less hypoglycemia.
- Near normal control of blood sugar levels.
- Bolus delivery options to match the type and amount of food.
- Predictable, readily available insulin.

Pumps cost about $6,000.00 and a year, and supplies cost about $2,000.00. Insurance coverage varies. Pump companies will be able to determine the coverage for pump therapy.

Resources

Medtronic MiniMed, Inc.
18000 Devonshire Street, Northridge, CA 91325-1219
1-800-646-4633
Website: www.minimed.com

Animas Corporation
590 Lancaster Avenue, Franger, PA 19355
1-877-937-7867
Website: www.animascorp.com

Deltec, Inc.
1265 Grey Fox Road
St. Paul, MN 55112
1-800-826-9703

Further Reading

The Insulin Pump Therapy Book: Insights from the Experts.
Edited by Linda Fredrickson, MA, RN, CDE from MiniMed
Technologies.

Outsmarting Diabetes. Richard S. Beaser, MD.

*Beating the Blood Sugar Blues: Problem Methods and Wisdom for
Controlling Hypoglycemia.* Thomas A. Lincoln, MD, and John
A. Eaddy, MD.

CHAPTER 9

Oral Medications

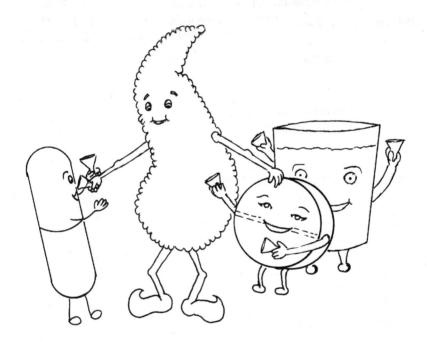

Oral Medications for Type 2 Diabetes

Your healthcare provider may prescribe medications if diet and exercise are not enough to keep your blood sugars in control. Remember, however, that even if you take medications for diabetes, diet and exercise are still necessary. You may need only one type of oral medication (not insulin), but if one does not work well, your may be prescribed one or two more. These medications work only if your beta cells are able to make some insulin. Also, with time, the effect of oral agents decreases. If this happens, you may need insulin.

How Do the Medications Work?

There are two major categories of medications: (1) oral hypoglycemic agents, which stimulate the production of insulin, and (2) oral antidiabetes agents, which include medications that decrease the amount of sugar that the liver makes, medications that help insulin to work better in the muscles and that lower insulin resistance, and medications that block the absorption of sugar from the intestines.

Remember: Even if you take medications for diabetes, diet and exercise are still necessary!

All medications have the possibility of side effects. Let your healthcare provider know if you have any of the following symptoms:

- Low blood sugar.
- Skin rash.
- Muscle aches.
- Loss of appetite.
- Metallic taste.
- Bloating, gas, or diarrhea.
- Nausea or vomiting.

Oral medications (pills) may be taken only once a day or three times a day. You may need only one type of medication or a combination of three or four medications. Be sure to take your pills as directed. Learn the name and dose of your medications. Write them down on a card and carry it with you.

Example of Card			
Date	Medication	Dose	Time

Drug Interaction Warning

Other medications can alter the effect of your diabetes medications. Please be sure to tell your healthcare provider about **all** of the pills, vitamins, herbs, and natural remedies that you are taking.

- If you miss a pill, do not add an extra one at your next dose time.
- Do not add pills if your blood sugar is high.
- If you are unable to eat, do not take your pills.
- Because all medications have the possibility of side effects, call your healthcare provider if you have nausea, muscle aches, fatigue, or a rash.

Resources

101 Medication Tips for People With Diabetes. Betsy A. Carlisle, PharmD, Lisa A. Kroon, PharmD, and Mary Anne Koda-Kimble, PharmD, CDE.

Additional Medication Information		
Medications (Generic Names)	Organ Affected	Action
Sulfonylureas Glimepiride Glipizide Glyburide Phenylalanine derivative Repaglinide Meglitinide Nateglinide	Pancreas	Stimulates insulin production and release
Biguanide Metformin	Liver	Decreases the amount of sugar made by the liver
Thiazolidinediones Pioglitazone Rosiglitazone	Muscle	Lowers insulin resistance and improves insulin action
Alpha-glucosidase inhibitors Acarbose Miglitol	Small intestine	Blocks the absorption of sugars

Important Facts to Remember

- Other drugs may interfere with the effectiveness of these medications.

- If you have liver or kidney disease or congestive heart disease, metformin may be contraindicated.

- Congestive heart failure may worsen with pioglitazone or rosiglitazone.

- Acarbose and miglitol are not recommended for those with intestinal disease or liver disease.

- Metformin (glucophage) must be stopped for 48 hours after any test using a contrast dye.

Oral Antidiabetic Agents (Inhibit a Rise in Blood Glucose)			
Medication	Brand Name	Dose (mg)	Possible Side Effects
Biguanide Metformin	Glucophage (XR)	500–2,500	Bloating, diarrhea, acids in blood
Thiazolidinediones			Edema, liver damage
Pioglitazone	Actose	15–45	
Rosiglitazone	Avandia	4–8	
Alpha-glucosidase inhibitors			Flatulence (gas), bloating
Miglitol	Glyset	25–300	
Acarbose	Precose	25–300	

Oral Hypoglycemic Agents (Lower Blood Glucose)			
Medication (Generic Name)	Brand Name	Dose (mg)	Possible Side Effects
Glimepiride	Amaryl	1–4	Hypoglycemia
Glipizide	Glucotrol	10–20	Hypoglycemia
Glyburide	DiaBeta, Micronase	1.5–20	Hypoglycemia
Nateglinide	Starlix	60–240	Hypoglycemia
Repaglinide	Prandin	1.5–16	Hypoglycemia

CHAPTER 10

Sick Day Management

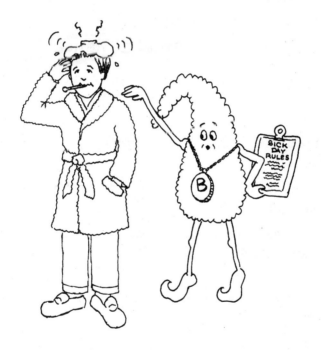

Your first sign of illness may be a high blood sugar that goes up hours before any other sign of illness is present. If you get a high blood sugar and don't know why, check again in a couple of hours and watch for any signs of illness.

Many kinds of illnesses can disrupt your blood glucose control. Viral colds or flu, infections, injuries, fever, vomiting, and diarrhea all increase your need for insulin. Emotional stress and surgery can also affect blood glucose levels. Learning to manage "sick days" at home can help you avoid hospitalization and can make you feel more comfortable until your illness has passed.

 If you get a high blood sugar and don't know why, check again in a couple of hours and watch for any signs of illness.

Sick Day Management at a Glance

1. **Never omit your insulin,** even if you can't eat. You may need additional insulin, but do not take additional oral hypoglycemic pills.

2. Test your blood sugar every 4 hours. If you need help, ask for it!

3. Replace meal carbohydrates with soups, Coke, Jell-O, sweet drinks, etc.

4. If you have Type 1 diabetes, test your urine for ketones every 4 hours if your blood sugar is over 250 mg.

5. Drink clear liquids (at least one-half cup every hour), and eat light foods if you can.

6. Rest. Do not exercise during an illness.

Call your doctor or healthcare provider if (1) you have an obvious infection, (2) your illness lasts longer than 2 days, (3) you have vomiting or diarrhea for more than 12 hours, (4) your blood sugar is over 400 mg on two con-secutive tests, (5) you have moderate to large urine ketones with a blood glucose level over 200 mg, (6) you feel very ill or experience pain, (7) you have extreme fatigue, shortness of breath, or dizziness, or (8) you have a high fever.

Correcting High Blood Sugars for People Who Take Insulin

When your blood sugar is high on sick days, adding extra fast-acting insulin can help you to stay out of trouble. We recommend the following methods for adding insulin on sick days:

1. Percentage Method

Most people will find this method easy to calculate. It is based on a person's total daily dose of insulin. Fast-acting insulin is used for the correction dose.

- Ten percent of the total daily dose is used to correct a high blood sugar.
- Twenty percent of the total daily dose is used to correct a high blood sugar plus ketones.

This may be given every 2 to 4 hours, but **not** at bedtime. If your total daily dose is 65 units, then 10% is 6.5 units (just put the decimal point in the middle), and 20% is 13 units (just double the 10% amount [6.5 units × 2 = 13 units]). Your healthcare provider will tell you when to add the 10% or 20%.

You may want to write your 10% or 20% dose for a quick reference: _____ × 10% = _____ units.

Example

One morning a young man awakens with a cold and sore throat. Because his blood sugar is 250 mg, he wants to correct his high blood sugar. He adds up all of his usual daily amounts of insulin:

Morning dose	20 units N
	4 units Humalog
Supper dose	6 units Humalog
Bedtime dose	10 units N
	40 units total daily dose

10% is 4 units and 20% is 8 units

This person now adds 4 units of Humalog to his breakfast dose. He will now take 20 units of N and 8 units of Humalog. At supper, his blood sugar is 300 mg, and his urine is positive for ketones. He takes an additional 20% of his total daily dose, or 8 units Humalog (20% of 40 = 8 units), and adds 8 units to his usual 6 units, which equals 14 units.

Always check with your healthcare provider before using this method.

2. Insulin Sensitivity Factor

The second method uses a formula called the "1,500 Rule." This is a system developed to estimate the drop in blood sugar that is caused by 1 unit of fast-acting insulin. This is also called the "insulin sensitivity factor." To calculate your sensitivity factor: add up your total daily dose of insulin (all insulins) and divide 1,500 by your total daily dose. The result is your insulin sensitivity factor.

Example

This person's total daily dose of insulin is 33 units. She awakens one morning with symptoms of a urinary tract infection. Her blood sugar is 223 mg.

- Divide 1,500 by the total daily dose: $1,500 \div 36 = 45$.

- The insulin sensitivity factor is 45 mg. One unit of fast-acting insulin will lower her blood sugar 45 mg.

- Because her target blood sugar is 90 mg, subtract the target blood sugar from the current blood sugar: $223 \text{ mg} - 90 \text{ mg} = 133 \text{ mg}$.

- She must lower her blood sugar 133 mg; thus, divide the sensitivity factor into the amount to be corrected: $133 \div 45 = 2.9$ or 3 units.

She adds 3 units of fast-acting insulin to her morning dose.

Many people are afraid to take insulin if they are unable to eat. The following guidelines will help you to stay in reasonable control and avoid hypoglycemia:

- When your blood sugar is low and you are unable to eat because of nausea and vomiting, take half of your usual intermediate insulin. Do not take your fast-acting insulin.

- Take your full dose of long-acting but no fast-acting insulin.

- Test your blood sugar in 2 to 4 hours.

- When your blood sugar goes up or you are able to eat, resume your usual dose of insulin.

Reminder

The fast-acting insulins are Humalog and Novolog. The intermediate insulins are N and L, and the long-acting insulins are U and Lantus.

A Sick Day Rules Diagram

Guidelines: Sick Day Management for the Insulin-Requiring Patient

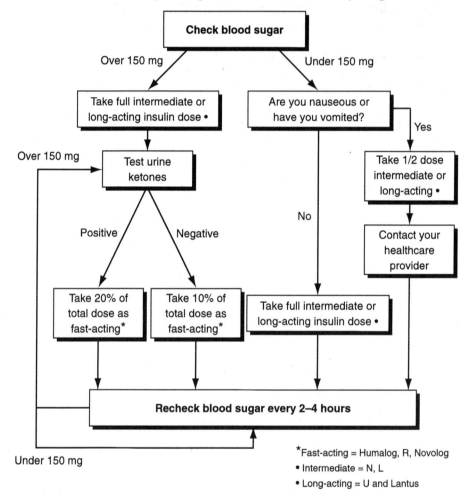

*Fast-acting = Humalog, R, Novolog
• Intermediate = N, L
• Long-acting = U and Lantus

If You Take Oral Hypoglycemic or Oral Antidiabetic Pills

Illness usually makes your blood sugar go up. However, sometimes if you are not eating, your blood sugar may go down. The diabetes pills that were taken hours before getting sick continue to work and may cause hypoglycemia (low blood sugar). If your blood sugar is low and you feel sweaty, shaky, weak, or dizzy, or if you look pale and feel numb and tingly, call your healthcare provider, call 911, or go immediately to an emergency room.

- It is important that you test your blood sugar at least twice a day when you are ill.

- Continue to take your diabetes medications.

- If you are vomiting, do not try to swallow pills. Wait until you can keep fluids down.

- Call your healthcare provider if your blood sugars are over 250 mg all day.

- Call your healthcare provider if your blood sugars are all under 100 mg and you have symptoms of hypoglycemia (low blood sugar).

Food for Sick Days

If you are too sick to follow your meal plan, try to replace carbohydrates with liquids or soft foods. Carbohydrates provide sugar so that the body does not have to burn fat for energy (burning fat produces ketones, which can be dangerous). Carbohydrates also prevent blood sugar from dropping too low. Small, frequent feedings may be easier for you to tolerate during an illness and can help your digestive system provide energy to your cells more quickly. Try to drink 4 ounces of clear liquids such as water, decaffeinated tea, apple juice, diet or regular soda, or sports drinks every hour.

If you can keep food down, but still have no appetite, try one-half cup of cream soup, one-half cup of cooked cereal, 1 cup of plain yogurt, Jell-O, one half of a banana, 1 scrambled egg, one-half cup of custard, or one-half cup of sherbet. Once you're feeling better, try adding toast or vanilla wafers and small amounts of food from your regular meal plan. Avoid spicy foods.

Nausea, Vomiting, and Diarrhea

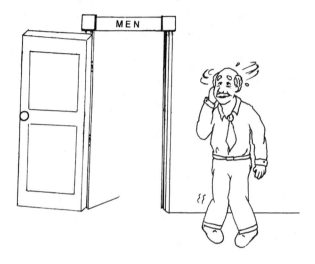

When you experience these symptoms, take small pieces of crushed ice or 1 to 2 ounces of regular cola or ginger ale (decarbonate by stirring) every 30 minutes. If you can keep this down, try adding soup or broth, tea, and clear juices. Soups and broths replace sodium and potassium, which are lost through vomiting and diarrhea.

Nonprescription Medicines for When You Are Sick

When people with diabetes get colds, allergies, and upset stomachs, over-the-counter medicines for these ailments may contain ingredients that raise or lower blood sugar or that mimic symptoms of high or low blood glucose. They may also increase blood pressure. Read the label before you purchase or use any over-the-counter medications. If there is a warning that people with diabetes should check with their doctors before using the product, do so. Some people with diabetes may be able to use the product, whereas others may not. Here are a few of the common over-the-counter medicines:

Coughs	Sugar-free cough syrups, expectorants, and cough suppressants
Sore Throat	Sugar-free lozenges, Tylenol, or aspirin
Congestion	Nasal sprays, Sudafed, Actifed
Allergies	Dimetapp Elixir, Benadryl, or any antihistamine
Diarrhea	Pepto-Bismol, Kaopectate, Donnagel, Imodium
Constipation	Enemas or suppositories, stool softeners, fiber therapy
Acid Stomach	Over-the-counter antacids—liquids or tablets
Nausea/Vomiting	Coke syrup, Emetrol (products contain sugar, but may be used in moderation, especially when one is not eating), Pepto-Bismol
Motion Sickness	Dramamine tablets, Scopolamine patch, Bonine
Skin Irritations	Cortisone creams, soothing powders
Minor Skin Infections	Antibiotic ointments or creams
Headaches	Tylenol, ibuprofen, aspirin
Muscle/Joint Pain	Aleve, ibuprofen, Icy Hot topical balm, capsaicin cream

Warnings

- Do not use appetite suppressants. Follow your diet and exercise plan to lose weight.

- Large amounts of aspirin may interact with diabetes medications, lowering blood sugar even more. Daily low-dose aspirin or a couple of aspirin now and then cause no harm for adults, however.

Caution

Cortisone shots for painful, inflamed joints will cause a tremendous increase in your blood sugar. This effect may last for days. Don't be alarmed. Call your healthcare provider for advice on how to handle these high blood sugars.

Notes

Extremely high blood sugars, left untreated, can lead to diabetic ketoacidosis or hyperosmolar hyperglycemic syndrome. Call your healthcare provider. The sooner you get help, the quicker you will get back into control. Keep your healthcare provider and pharmacy phone numbers near your phone. Keep these sick-day supplies on hand: both sugar-free and regular soda and clear liquids; Tylenol, aspirin, or ibuprofen (do not take ibuprofen if you have kidney problems); cold/flu medications that your healthcare provider has approved; a thermometer; and antinausea medications.

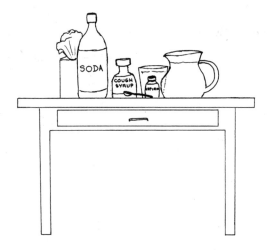

CHAPTER 11

Foot Care, Skin Care, and Dental Hygiene

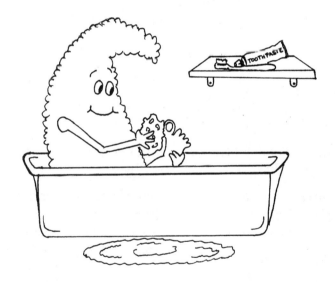

Preventing Problems

People with long-term diabetes may be prone to skin and foot problems. People who have had diabetes for a short time, children and teens, and those who have no diabetic complications simply need to follow healthy common sense hygiene and caution.

Foot Problems

If you have good sensation in your feet and have no circulation problems, you may skip this section. Just follow common sense to keep your feet healthy. If you get a cut or blister, clean it and cover it until it heals. People who have had poorly controlled diabetes for a long time or people with diabetes that has gone undetected for a long time may develop serious foot problems.

Why Does This Happen?

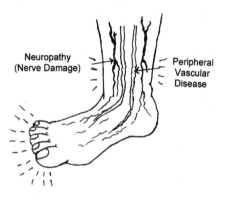

Neuropathy
(Nerve Damage)

Peripheral
Vascular
Disease

Typically, there is a combination of two problems: peripheral vascular disease and neuropathy.

- Peripheral vascular disease means "poor circulation." Poor blood circulation to and from your feet slows the healing process and limits your ability to fight infection. If you have this problem, your feet will feel cold and may cramp, and the pulses in your feet may be hard to feel. Even small injuries will not heal and may turn into an ulcer.

- Neuropathy, or "nerve damage," lessens your ability to feel pain, heat, and cold. This puts you at high risk for foot injuries. With this problem, your first sign may be numbness and tingling in your toes. Sharp, shooting, stabbing pain can be felt when you put your feet up in the late afternoon and evening or when you go to bed. Damaged nerves lessen the ability of your feet to produce natural moisture, resulting in dry feet that crack and peel.

Because of nerve damage, you may see changes in the shape of your foot over time. A high arch, protruding ball of your foot, and hammertoes can occur. Calluses and ulcers form on the pressure areas created by the "retracted" foot.

Calluses

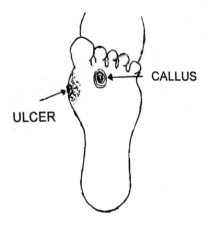

Calluses are caused by the constant rubbing of shoes over a pressure area. Use a pumice stone or have a podiatrist remove this thick, hard skin.

Ulcers

Ulcers can form over any pressure points on your foot. Constant pressure breaking down layers of skin causes ulcers, which are open sores or holes in the skin. The most common place for these to develop is the ball of the foot. If the ulcer goes as deep as the bone, the bone can also get infected. This requires surgery to remove the infected bone or foot.

How Can I Prevent Foot Ulcers?

If you have both poor circulation and nerve damage, you are at high risk for foot ulcers. Prevention of pressure points and skin breakdown along with daily self foot checks can save your feet.

Tips

- Do not cut your own toenails if you have nerve damage, poor circulation, poor eyesight, or difficulty reaching them. Get help or see a podiatrist.

- Extra depth shoes and molded shoes might be needed to prevent pressure points, calluses, and ulcers.

- If you smoke—stop! Smoking increases the risk for amputations.

- Padded or double socks reduce callus buildups.

- Tie shoes can be adjusted for feet that swell in the afternoon.

- Love your feet? Don't neglect them!

Charcot's Foot

This condition starts with severe nerve damage to the feet. The bones become thin, and muscles in the foot become weak. Normal walking can cause a fracture that may cause no discomfort or minimal discomfort. Swelling and redness may be the only sign. Sometimes people with this problem continue to walk on the injured foot, causing joint damage, which cannot be reversed. The foot is left large and deformed as the joint fuses in a bulging position.

If you are at risk for this problem, wear supportive shoes with a molded insert. Avoid high foot impact activities. Use caution when you step off curbing or stairs, and call your healthcare provider if you notice any swelling of your foot.

Early casting and no weight bearing lessen the deformity.

Foot Care Dos and Don'ts

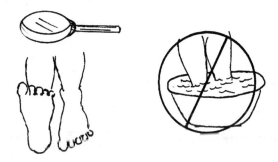

DOs & DON'Ts OF FOOT CARE

It is good to do the following:

- Check your feet daily for red spots, bruises, cuts, blisters, and dryness or cracks in the skin. Use a mirror to see the bottoms of your feet. Don't forget under and between toes. Press gently and feel for tenderness or hot spots—this may indicate injury even if you feel no pain.

- Every day, wash your feet in warm—not hot—water (check water on wrist or elbow) and mild soap. Dry them thoroughly, especially between the toes.

- If the skin on your feet is dry, apply a lanolin-based cream (but not between the toes). If your feet perspire a lot, use talcum powder. Shake out your shoes before putting them on. Feel the inside of your shoes to check for cracks or torn, loose linings that could irritate your feet.

- Wear good-fitting, soft shoes and clean socks. Smooth out wrinkles in socks. Choose new shoes carefully (a proper fit is more important than style) and break them in slowly (only 1 to 2 hours per day). Check for red pressure areas when you remove your shoes and socks.

- Avoid foot injuries by wearing shoes or slippers around the house and water shoes at the beach or pool.
- Wear insulated boots to keep feet warm on cold days.
- Trim toenails after bathing when they are soft. Cut toenails straight across and then file the corners to the contour of your toe. If you can't see them well or reach them easily, have someone do this for you.
- Buff calluses with a pumice stone.
- Avoid high-impact exercise if you have poor sensation in your feet.

Don't do the following:

- Dig under toenails or try to cut ingrown toenails.
- Put hot water bottles, heating pads, or items heated in a microwave on your feet.
- Soak your feet (this dries out natural oils).
- Cut corns or calluses with a razor or use corn pads or corn medication.
- Wear shoes that are too tight or worn out or tight socks that cut off circulation, as shoes that don't fit well cause blisters and calluses.

Call your healthcare provider if you have any of the following:

- A puncture wound, any foot injury that does not heal, or any pus from cuts.
- Red spots (even if there is no pain) under corns and calluses.
- Ingrown or thick toenails, corns, or calluses that are difficult to care for.

First Aid for Foot Injuries

You may feel no pain when you injure your foot, but that doesn't mean you can ignore the injury.

- Wash the injury with mild soap and dry thoroughly.
- Then apply a mild antiseptic ointment or cream.
- Do not use iodine, Epsom salts, or boric acid.
- If a bandage is necessary, use a small gauze pad and nonallergic tape (regular tape can irritate your skin).
- Rest with the injured foot up for 20 minutes several times a day.
- Call your healthcare provider if the injury has not improved in 2 to 3 days or if it is infected.

Sock News

Special socks are made for special feet. For sweaty feet, polypropylene wicks away moisture. Doubling fabric socks helps to prevent blisters and calluses. Thick-cushioned socks help prevent pressure areas. Wool socks warm cold feet.

Common Skin Problems

Dryness

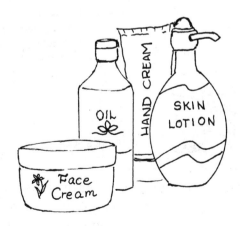

There are three common causes for dry skin. First, long-term diabetes may have affected the body's ability to produce natural oils, which keep skin soft and supple. Second, poorly controlled diabetes keeps a person constantly dehydrated (not enough fluid in the body). Third, heredity is a factor.

What Can I Do for My Dry Skin?

Use a lanolin-base cream applied to dry skin after a shower or bath. The cream will hold in the moisture. Bath oils are good also but may be very slippery. If you have a buildup of thick, dry skin, you may need a prescription lotion or cream. Several creams and lotions are made specifically for people with diabetes.

Rashes

A skin irritant, an allergic reaction to medications, or viruses can cause rashes. Contact your healthcare provider if you develop a rash that does not clear up in a few days.

Fungal Infections

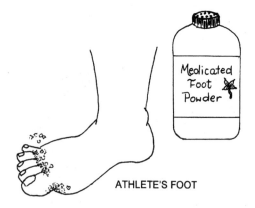

ATHLETE'S FOOT

Fungal infections occur more frequently in people with un-controlled diabetes. Yeast loves to grow in warm, moist areas such as the groin, underarms, perineum, the vagina, and the breasts. The excess sugar from uncontrolled diabetes feeds the yeast buds. This infection is itchy and red and has a cheesy white discharge. Antifungal creams work, but the infection will come back with high blood sugars. Toenails and sometimes fingernails can become infected. Nails become thick, yellow, and brittle and are difficult to trim.

Medications are available for treating nail fungi. They are expensive and have to be taken intermittently for 3 months, and it may take up to 1 year to see the final results. People who have liver problems cannot take this medication. Several new topical solutions are available and have worked for some. Mild irritation around the nail may occur from this topical solution.

Athlete's Foot

Athlete's foot affects many people, including those with diabetes. This fungal infection causes itchiness, tiny blisters, or scaly, dry skin. It is often found between the toes. Athlete's foot is very contagious and can be caught from contact with fungus that is found on bathroom floors, public locker rooms, and showers. Because the broken skin may lead to other infections, it is best to treat it quickly. Use antifungal creams or powders daily on your feet, socks, and shoes. Rotate shoes so that they can dry between uses. Prescription creams may be needed for more severe cases. Prevent athlete's foot by wearing bath shoes in public showers and bathhouses.

Other Skin Infections

People with uncontrolled diabetes are prone to infections because high blood sugars reduce the effectiveness of bacteria-fighting cells, and bacteria grows rapidly when more sugar is around. Even a small cut may progress to a deep, open sore. Carbuncles and boils may become a serious problem. Antibiotic creams, ointments, and pills are used to treat infections.

How Do I Know If Infection Is Present?

The first sign of an infection is a high blood sugar level. Other signs of infection include pain, fever, redness, warmth over and around the site, swelling, and possibly discharge. Don't hesitate to call your healthcare provider if you have any of these signs. Preventing foot, skin, and dental problems begins with good diabetes control. Even if you have had diabetes for a very long time and have experienced some problems, you'll want to learn as much as possible so that you can prevent further problems. Diabetic dermopathy appears as red or brown scaly spots on shins and ankles. Almost 60% of people with long-term diabetes have these lesions. They are harmless, and no treatment is available. "Diabetic sclerosis" is the hardening and thickening of skin, especially seen on the fingers, hands, toes, and across the upper back and shoulders. The skin will look shiny and feel waxy. It can cause an achy and stiff feeling. It is seen only in people with long-term diabetes. No treatment is available, but ibuprofen or aspirin may ease pain.

Dental Care

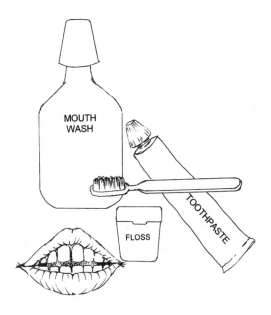

```
┌─────────────────────────────────────────────┐
│              Dr. Goodgum, D.M.D.              │
│                                               │
│  M _____   │
│            HAS AN APPOINTMENT ON:             │
│                                               │
│  _____  │
│   DAY          MONTH              DATE        │
│                                               │
│  AT _____ A.M. _____ P.M.       │
│                                               │
│        PLEASE GIVE 24 HOURS NOTICE            │
│        IF UNABLE TO KEEP APPOINTMENT          │
└─────────────────────────────────────────────┘
```

People with uncontrolled diabetes are more prone to cavities and gum infections and may heal more slowly after dental surgery. High blood sugars slow healing while supporting an overgrowth of mouth bacteria. This can be controlled by first working toward good diabetes control and then doing the following:

- Brush your teeth at least twice a day.

- See your dentist for regular checkups and cleanings.

- Call your dentist if you have any bleeding from gums, mouth sores, or a painful tooth.

- Stop smoking.

Further Reading

101 Foot Care Tips for People with Diabetes. Jesse H. Ahroni, PhD, ARNP, CDE.

CHAPTER 12

Complications

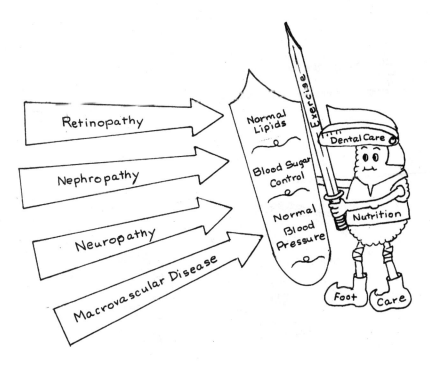

Complications

All people with Type 1 and Type 2 diabetes are at risk for
complications, although they may not appear for many
years. In fact, evidence is available that with good blood
sugar control and normalized blood pressure and blood fat
levels, complications can be prevented or minimized.
Evidence shows that some early complications can be
reversed with good control. Do all that you can to prevent

complications. The old saying "an ounce of prevention is worth a pound of cure" is especially true here.

You may already have some diabetes complications. The length of time that you have had diabetes, genetics, and your level of control over the years influence your stage of complications. Even if you have some complications, it's never too late to slow the progress of these problems.

 An ounce of prevention is worth a pound of cure.

Eye Diseases

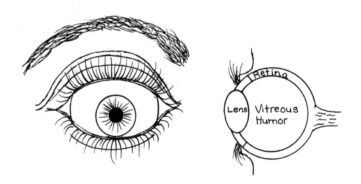

Diabetes can affect (1) the **lens** of the eye, which focuses light reflected from objects; (2) the **retina,** where images are formed and translated into electric impulses for interpretation by the brain; and (3) the **vitreous humor,** a clear jelly-like substance through which light passes from the lens to the retina.

Cataracts and Blurred Vision

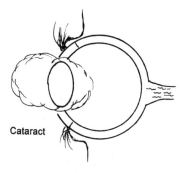

Cataract

Cataracts are clouding of the normally clear lens. A cataract develops over years and causes blurred vision when a large part of the lens becomes cloudy. Causes of cataracts include aging, eye injuries, disease, heredity, and birth defects. **Senile cataracts** are a common eye problem among the older population. Poor diabetes control can hasten the formation of senile cataracts. **Metabolic cataracts** are sometimes found in younger people with diabetes. Surgical removal of the lens treats both types. Eyeglasses, contact lenses, or intraocular lens implants restore vision after surgery.

Blurred vision is caused by changes in the blood sugar. As blood sugar increases, more sugar and water move into the lens, causing it to swell. When the blood sugar goes back down, even more water rushes into the lens, causing greater swelling. When the blood sugar stabilizes, the lens will also stabilize. Often people think that they need a change in their eyeglass prescription.

Glaucoma, the inability of fluid to flow normally through the eye, is three times more prevalent in people with diabetes. This causes an increase of fluid and pressure inside the eye. If left untreated or undetected, glaucoma can cause blindness.

Diabetic Retinopathy

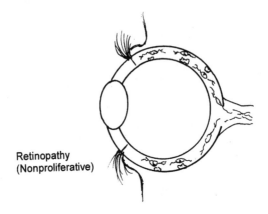

Retinopathy
(Nonproliferative)

Diabetic retinopathy is a deterioration of the small blood vessels that nourish the retina. Although diabetic retinopathy is a serious cause of blindness, only a small percentage of persons with diabetic retinopathy lose their sight. Two forms of diabetic retinopathy exist: nonproliferative retinopathy and proliferative retinopathy.

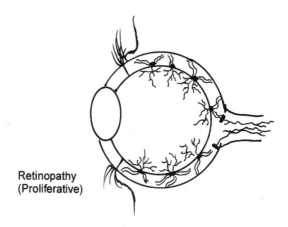

Retinopathy
(Proliferative)

Nonproliferative retinopathy, also known as background retinopathy, is an early stage of retinopathy that is free of any symptoms. Blood vessels within the retina develop tiny bulges (microaneurysms) that leak fluid, causing swelling and forming deposits (exudates). The macula (the part of the retina where central vision occurs) becomes swollen, resulting in distorted vision. Good diabetes control may slow the progress of retinopathy. In some cases, this may progress to proliferative retinopathy.

Proliferative retinopathy develops when retinal vessels become blocked and fragile nerve blood vessels grow on the retina and into the vitreous humor. If left untreated, these tiny, fragile vessels rupture, bleeding into the vitreous humor and blocking light from the retina. When a rupture or hemorrhage occurs, it may look like black spots, a spider web, or a glob. This may disappear in 3 to 6 months, but scar tissue and possibly some loss of vision are left. Hemorrhages close to the macula area cause a greater loss of vision.

The ruptured blood vessels form scar tissue that may tighten and pull on the retina, eventually detaching it from the back of the eye. This is called retinal detachment and may look like a dark streak or a curtain being pulled across the eye. **An urgent visit to your ophthalmologist may save your vision.** Regular eye visits to your ophthalmologist can spot early problems. Your ophthalmologist can treat you with laser surgery called **photocoagulation** before tiny blood vessels rupture and bleed into the vitreous humor. Laser therapy is the treatment for proliferative retinopathy. A finely focused laser beam is aimed at the retina to burn out proliferative vessels and to lessen the demand for new vessel formation.

Vitrectomy

When massive bleeding into the vitreous humor has occurred, a vitrectomy can be performed. In this surgical procedure, the bloody vitreous humor is removed and replaced with clear, sterile fluids, restoring vision. This surgery is not without risks, however.

To minimize the risk of diabetic retinopathy, (1) keep your blood sugar level in good control, (2) maintain normal blood pressure, and (3) see an ophthalmologist for a complete eye exam at least once a year or as recommended.

Kidney Disease

The kidneys filter waste products from the blood, rid the body of excess water, and eliminate certain chemicals. Needed chemicals, proteins, and red and white blood cells remain in the blood stream. The kidneys produce about a quart of urine every day to maintain the body's fluid balance.

Diabetic Nephropathy

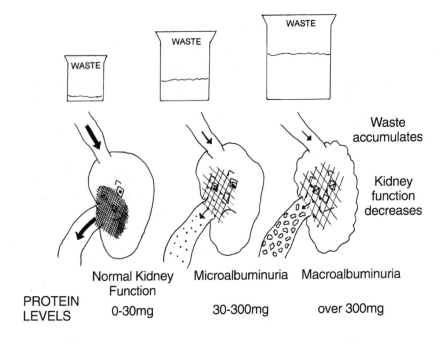

	Normal Kidney Function	Microalbuminuria	Macroalbuminuria
PROTEIN LEVELS	0-30mg	30-300mg	over 300mg

Waste accumulates

Kidney function decreases

Diabetic nephropathy is a complication of long-term diabetes that results in damage and thickening to the bundles of capillaries that form the kidneys' filtering system. Diabetic nephropathy develops in stages over many years. Kidney filtering becomes less efficient, and certain proteins leak out; waste products are not filtered and build up in the blood. Microscopic amounts of protein (microalbuminuria) in the urine may be the first sign of nephropathy. Later signs include high blood pressure, weight gain from fluid retention, fatigue, and feeling ill. Kidney function tests help to determine the degree of kidney damage.

The tests include a spot urine test for microalbuminuria, 24-hour urine for protein, and a blood test for waste products called creatinine and blood urea nitrogen. Blood tests may not show any changes until more than 80% of the kidneys are damaged.

When kidneys fail completely you may feel very tired and have nausea, a poor appetite, and weight loss. Treatments for kidney failure include hemodialysis, peritoneal dialysis, and kidney transplants.

To minimize the risk of diabetic nephropathy:

- Keep your blood sugar level in control.

- Maintain normal blood pressure. Don't forget to take medications your doctor has prescribed for high blood pressure. Experts suggest the use of special drugs called angiotensin-converting enzyme inhibitors.

- Follow the specific diet that your healthcare provider and dietitian recommended.

Urinary Tract Infections

Urinary tract infections can develop in persons with uncontrolled or controlled diabetes. Symptoms include excessive urination, a burning sensation with urination, lower back pain, and fever. If untreated, the infection travels up the ureters to the kidney, possibly causing permanent damage. Women are more likely to develop urinary tract infections. Prompt treatment with antibiotics that your healthcare provider prescribed is essential. Remember to take the pills for the period prescribed, even if your symptoms go away.

Nerve Damage (Neuropathy)

Nearly 70% of people with diabetes have some degree of nerve damage or neuropathy. Neuropathy occurs in people with Type 1 and Type 2 diabetes. Constant high blood sugars cause metabolic changes that destroy both nerve fibers (axons) and the fatty insulation that surrounds them (myelin). Damaged nerves do not transmit correct signals, resulting in a loss of sensation, hypersensation, pain, muscle weakness, and loss of some body functions. There are three types of nerves: sensory nerves, which tell us how something feels; motor nerves, which tell your body to move; and autonomic nerves, which control the automatic body functions such as heart rate.

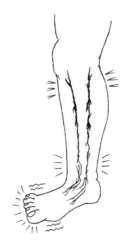

Sensory nerve damage causes loss of feeling, resulting in hypersensation and pain. It starts in the toes and moves up to the feet and legs. When it reaches the knees, it may also be found in the hands. If you have this, you will have numbness, tingling, burning, stabbing pains, and cramping, which are worse at night. Your skin may be so sensitive that pressure from clothing feels painful. The greatest danger is foot injury and ulcers (see Chapter 11).

Treatment

- Control of blood sugar is important.

- Medications can control pain.

- Topical creams containing capsaicin (a pepper derivative) may provide some relief.

- Alternative treatments, which have no scientific data regarding effectiveness, have been used. Patches containing the medication lidocaine and acupuncture have been successful in some patients.

Motor nerve damage causes muscle weakness. If you have this you may not be able to have strength enough for everyday chores and activities. You may have difficulty opening jars, grasping items, or walking.

Autonomic nerve damage affects multiple body systems.

- Damage to heart nerves causes a rapid resting heart rate.

- Damage to bladder nerves causes incomplete emptying of urine and difficulty urinating, leading to bladder infections and a large, baggy bladder.

- Postural hypotension (a drop in blood pressure when sitting up or standing quickly) causes dizziness, light-headedness, and possibly fainting, which are caused by damage to nerves that regulate blood vessels.

- When nerves to the stomach are affected, food is delayed in passing. As it sits there, it can cause nausea, vomiting, and bloating. This is called gastroparesis.

- Damage to intestinal nerves can cause "diabetic diarrhea," alternating with constipation. Diarrhea may occur during the night without warning.

- When nerves to the skin are damaged, abnormal sweating and blood vessel constriction occur. Profuse sweating above the waist with no sweating of feet and constricting blood vessels in warm temperatures may be signs of this problem. Sweating heavily after large meals is most likely from a combination of damaged nerves.

- Men may experience erectile dysfunction from damage to nerves that control erections. Damage to blood vessels in the penis and poor diabetes control make the problem worse.

- Loss of normal warning of low blood sugar (hypoglycemic unawareness).

How Can I Prevent or Lessen Nerve Damage?

- Keep blood sugars as close to normal as possible.

- Drink less alcohol, as too much alcohol can accelerate neuropathy.

Blood Vessels

Large Blood Vessels: Macrovascular Disease

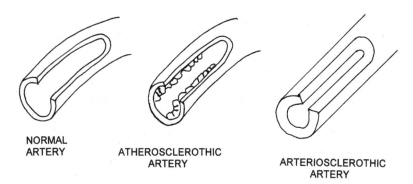

NORMAL
ARTERY

ATHEROSCLEROTHIC
ARTERY

ARTERIOSCLEROTHIC
ARTERY

Macrovascular disease refers to changes in the medium- to large-sized blood vessels. The blood vessel walls thicken and become hard and nonelastic (arteriosclerosis). Blood vessels also become clogged with mounds of plaque deposited from cholesterol and triglycerides (atherosclerosis). High blood sugars cause platelets in the blood to stick and clump on the plaque. Eventually, the flow of blood may be blocked. Three types of this disease are as follows:

- **Peripheral vascular disease** refers to diseased blood vessels that supply the legs and feet. If blood flow is only partially interrupted, cramps, weakness, "charley horses," or pain in the legs when walking (claudication) may result. Poor healing of foot injuries is evident (see Chapter 11). A completely blocked artery will cause severe pain, and the leg will become cold and pale. Treatments include replacing the diseased artery surgically or opening the blood vessel by compressing plaque against the artery wall (angioplasty).

Heart

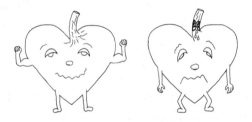

- **Coronary artery disease** refers to diseased heart arteries. Cramping and angina can occur when blood flow is decreased. Complete blockage of an artery results in myocardial infarction (MI), or heart attack. Symptoms of angina and heart attack include chest pressure, cramping, a heavy feeling in the chest, shortness of breath, and extreme fatigue. **Don't delay. Immediate treatment saves lives and starts damage control!** Treatments include medications, coronary bypass surgery, and angioplasty. Sometimes there are very few symptoms warning of a heart attack. Overwhelming fatigue and shortness of breath may be the only symptoms. This is called a silent MI (heart attack).

Brain

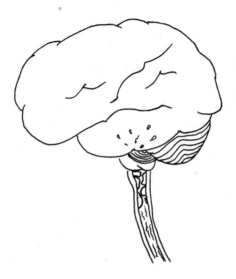

- **Cerebral vascular disease** refers to diseased arteries in the brain. Partial blockage may result in temporary reductions of blood supply to a part of the brain (transient ischemic attacks). A complete loss of blood supply to an area of the brain due to clogging or breaking of a blood vessel results in a cerebral vascular accident (stroke). Symptoms include lightheadedness, dizziness, a loss of ability to speak, slurred speech, confusion, and inappropriate behavior. Treatments include medications, coronary bypass surgery, and angioplasty.

If you experience symptoms of any form of macrovascular disease, go to a hospital emergency room at once.

Risk Factors

The most important risk factor for macrovascular disease (clogged arteries) is heredity. However, other factors may accelerate this problem.

Risk Factor	Treatment
Diabetes	Control blood sugar
High blood pressure	Medication to lower blood pressure
Obesity	Reduce weight
Inactivity	Exercise
High cholesterol and triglycerides	Healthy eating—low fat
Smoking	Stop smoking

To Minimize the Risk of Macrovascular Disease

- Keep your blood sugar level in good control.
- Maintain normal blood pressure. If necessary, don't forget to take medication for high blood pressure.
- If necessary, try to reduce your weight.
- Reduce fats and cholesterol in your diet.
- Exercise in moderation, after consulting with your healthcare provider.
- Do not smoke.
- See your doctor regularly.

Never give up hope. Much of the research is focusing on not only the prevention of complications but also the successful treatment of complications.

Complications	Organ	Function Affected
Small blood vessels		
Retinopathy	Eyes	Sight
Nephropathy	Kidneys	Elimination of waste
Neuropathy		
Peripheral	Nerves	Sensation & motor function
Autonomic	Heart	Rate
	Bladder	Difficulty emptying
	Blood vessels	Unstable blood pressure
	Stomach	Slow emptying
	Intestines	Constipation/diarrhea
	Skin	Sweating
Large blood vessels		
Coronary	Heart	Circulation
Peripheral	Legs and feet, brain	Circulation

Further Reading

The Uncomplicated Guide to Diabetes Complications. Edited by Marvin E. Levin, MD, and Michael A. Pfiefer, MD.

CHAPTER 13

Diabetes and the Family

Special concerns of families who are coping with diabetes are addressed here. Part I focuses on the special needs of women with diabetes during pregnancy. Part II provides advice for parents of children with diabetes. Part III gives information for school personnel who have contact with students who have diabetes. Part IV gives information on how to support a family member.

Part I: Pregnancy

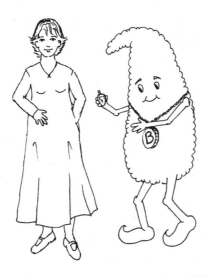

Women with Type 1 and Type 2 diabetes can have safe, healthy pregnancies. The risk to mother and baby can be kept to a minimum with excellent blood sugar control before and during pregnancy. Pregnancy, however, will demand more time and attention to your diabetes and will be expensive.

Plan Before Pregnancy

Before you become pregnant, try to get the best blood sugar possible and target your hemoglobin A1c to 6%. Your doctor will give you a complete physical examination and check for any complications. Meet with an obstetrician that has experience working with women who have diabetes and who will work well with your diabetes healthcare team, which may include a diabetes educator, a diabetologist, a dietitian, and a neonatologist. Meet with a nutritionist and attain a healthy weight. Establish an exercise program. If you take pills for diabetes, you will need to change to insulin injections. Stop smoking and drinking alcohol before pregnancy begins, as these are both harmful to babies.

During Pregnancy

First Trimester

During the first 6 weeks, the baby's organs are formed. Uncontrolled diabetes during this time increases the risk of birth defects. Mild to moderate—not strenuous—exercise is recommended. Your blood sugars may decrease during this time because the developing baby uses up a lot of energy. You may even have to lower your insulin doses if you experience nausea and vomiting. Carry fast-acting sugar to treat low blood sugars quickly. An ultrasound may be ordered to date your pregnancy.

Second Trimester

During this time, your baby continues to grow and develop, and you will gain weight. The increase in weight and hormones produced during pregnancy increases your need for insulin, especially between the 24th and 26th weeks. It is important to increase your insulin when needed so that your baby does not get exposed to high blood sugars, as these sugars go directly to the baby. The baby's pancreas works fine and pours out insulin. Extra sugar and lots of insulin cause big babies (macrosomia). No woman wants to deliver a 10- to 12-pound baby! You will have a comprehensive ultrasound test and a fetal echocardiogram to screen for birth defects.

Third Trimester

Your baby's organs are fully formed. Now the baby grows rapidly and your insulin requirements continue to increase. You and your healthcare team will start to plan for delivery. You will have more ultrasound tests to follow the baby's growth, and you may also have a nonstress test to check the baby's response and movements and possibly an amniocentesis to check for the baby's lung maturity.

Delivery Time

- To be safe, obstetricians usually set delivery dates slightly before the due date.

- Labor may be induced or a cesarian section scheduled.

- You and your baby will be carefully monitored during labor.

- Your blood sugars are best kept under 120 mg/dl.

- Once your baby is delivered, you will need only about half of your prepregnancy insulin dose.

- Discuss with your healthcare provider how to prepare for this dramatic decrease in insulin requirement.

- Your blood sugars will be closely monitored after delivery to watch for hypoglycemia.
- Your baby will also be closely monitored for hypoglycemia.

After Delivery

- You may continue to require less insulin for 3 to 4 weeks after delivery, and your blood sugars may be unpredictable because of hormonal fluctuations.
- If you have Type 2 diabetes, you may not require any insulin or medications for a month or more after delivery.
- If you are breastfeeding, you may experience drops in your blood sugar when you nurse your baby. Prepare quick, healthy snacks to eat or drink when nursing to avoid this problem.

What Are Some of the Risks of Pregnancy?

- An increase in established eye and kidney complications.
- Generalized edema (usually late in pregnancy).
- Hydramnios (excessive amounts of amniotic fluid).
- Preeclampsia (elevated blood pressure, protein in urine, and swelling of hands and feet).

What Are the Risks for My Baby?

- Statistics show that there is a 6% to 12% risk of birth defects for babies who are born to women with diabetes who have had "average" blood sugar control.
- The risk of birth defects drops to 2% to 3% when excellent blood sugar control is achieved before and during pregnancy.
- There is a greater risk for having large babies, weighing 9.5 pounds or more, when blood sugars are above normal, especially in the second and third trimesters.

- Your baby may have low blood sugar (hypoglycemia) after birth. If your blood sugars have been over normal during pregnancy or just before delivery, your baby's pancreas is revved up to produce a lot of insulin. After birth, your baby will continue to make high levels of insulin but is no longer receiving extra sugar from you. Intravenous glucose is used to treat this.

- Jaundice is caused when the baby's liver is not developed enough to take care of the disposal of extra red blood cells that your baby needed to make before delivery. The breakdown product of these red blood cells and bilirubin remains in the blood and colors the baby's skin yellow. Special lights are used to treat this condition.

What Is the Chance That My Baby Will Get Diabetes?

If you have Type 1 diabetes, the risk of your child developing diabetes is 2% to 7%. If the baby's father has Type 1 diabetes, the risk increases slightly. For Type 2 diabetes, the risk in a lifetime is greater; however, obesity is an important factor. Diabetes is extremely rare in babies.

Gestational Diabetes

Gestational diabetes is diagnosed during pregnancy, usually during the 24th to 26th week of pregnancy. It occurs more frequently in women who are overweight or have a family history of diabetes. After delivery, the majority of these women no longer have diabetes but are at greater risk of developing diabetes in the future. Treatment of gestational diabetes always begins with a meal plan and exercise; insulin is introduced only if the meal plan and exercise regimen fail to keep blood sugars in a normal range. The goal is to normalize before- and after-meal blood sugars. If you are diagnosed with gestational diabetes, your obstetrician may expand your healthcare team to include a diabetes educator, a diabetologist, a dietitian, and a neonatologist. The American Diabetes Association and the

American Academy of Obstetrics and Gynecology do not recommend the use of oral antidiabetic agents during pregnancy because of safety issues.

Further Reading

Diabetes and Pregnancy, What to Expect. Available from the American Diabetes Association bookstore: 1-800-232-6733.

Gestational Diabetes. Available from the American Diabetes Association bookstore: 1-800-232-6733.

Part II: Advice for Parents of Children with Diabetes

When you learned that your child has diabetes, you may have experienced disbelief, grief, and guilt. Maybe you asked why did this happen to my child or said, "It's not fair!" You must come to grips with these feelings so that you can learn the tasks and techniques of diabetes control. Your entire family needs to make adjustments to your child's condition. How you deal with and accepts diabetes affects the way that your child deals with and accept diabetes. The more you know about diabetes, the better equipped you are to help your child. A number of books are available that discuss children with diabetes.

Goals for Children with Diabetes

- Normal growth and development.
- Optimal blood sugar control.
- Minimal episodes of hypoglycemia or prolonged hyperglycemia and diabetic ketoacidosis.
- Good psychosocial adjustment.

As a parent, you are naturally anxious, but it's up to you to help your child accept his or her diabetes with a minimum amount of stress. The American Diabetes Association and the Juvenile Diabetes Foundation can be of great help. Your local affiliate may have a support group. Other parents who have faced the same problem and have learned to cope with it are more than willing to share ideas and advice. You must learn to protect without dominating and to supervise while encouraging self-efficacy. Work with your child for the best control, but remember that "ideal" blood sugars are not always possible.

Diabetes threatens your child's self-image and self-esteem. Be understanding and supportive. Try to avoid unnecessary anxiety about "cheating." You don't want to cause guilt feelings or make your child think he or she is "bad." Children who think that they are bad may act accordingly. Help your child plan ahead. No child should be expected to assume complete responsibility for diabetes control at too early of an age. Ultimately, however, eating properly, injecting insulin, testing blood sugar, and planning exercise will be the child's responsibility. Maturity, independence, self-control, and self-esteem will grow as your child learns to care for himself or herself.

A child with diabetes is a child first and a person with diabetes second. Your child, like all others, needs to grow physically, socially, and emotionally. He or she needs alert parents who are relaxed, knowledgeable, and tolerant, and who listen well and are able to accept help in the growing process. Feelings of guilt and resentment lead to problems between spouses and between parents and children. Your child's diabetes is a challenge that your entire family must face together. It is not a punishment for anyone's actions.

 Your child is a child first and a person with diabetes second. He or she needs you to be relaxed, knowledgeable, and tolerant.

Pitfalls for Parents

An overanxious parent creates an overanxious child who is too dependent. By doing everything for your child, you deny him or her the self-control and self-confidence that are necessary for an independent life.

An overindulgent parent feels that dietary restrictions and daily injections are too much for a child to handle and thus offers special treats while providing little discipline. Children of overindulgent parents may grow up under the impression that they are incompetent—incapable of coping with their own problems—which reinforces feelings of inadequacy.

A parent who is a perfectionist may achieve good diabetes management in early childhood through discipline, but there are risks. The child may feel guilty about poor blood sugar test results and may even alter a result to obtain parental approval. During adolescence, children of perfectionist parents may rebel against both their parents and their diabetes care programs.

A parent who is indifferent may force his or her child to seek attention through rebellion by "cheating" on the diet or by skipping insulin injections. Children of indifferent parents may become depressed because of the lack of discipline, support, and supervision in their lives. They also have a higher frequency of hospitalization.

The Parent's Role

Your role as the parent of a child with diabetes will change as your child grows. Every child is different, of course, but there are some general guidelines that you can follow at each stage. These are some things that you should remember no matter the age of your child. Accept your child. Love, teach, guide, and discipline just as you would if diabetes were not a factor. Do not overprotect or overindulge. Accept your child's diabetes without guilt. Learn all that you can about diabetes to help you to overcome your fears and anxieties. Remember that you cannot control your child's diabetes by overcontrolling your child.

Years 0 Through 7

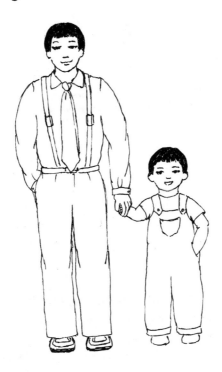

During early childhood, the parent has full responsibility for all aspects of diabetes care. It's important to involve the child at an early age, however. Offer some choices, such as picking a spot to inject or selecting from which finger to get the drop of blood. Remember that parental approval is important at this age: Be sure that you describe blood test results as high, low, or normal—not as good or bad.

Years 7 Through 12

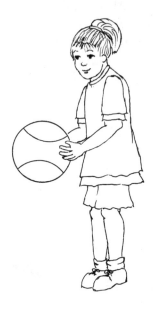

Although the parent continues to take major responsibility, during this period, the child can take over blood sugar testing and insulin injections some of the time. By age 12, most children can manage their own injections, but parents must be vigilant and remind them if they forget. Children who are away at school or who are playing with friends most of the day must assume partial responsibility for dietary control. Participation in self-care at an early age encourages the child to become independent and self-reliant.

Try not to be rigid. Children need to learn that a reasonable compromise is all right for parties and special occasions. There is no reason for them to feel "different." A serving of birthday cake and ice cream may elevate blood sugar, but the emotional value of participating with other children is also important. Cover extra food with a few units of Humalog or regular insulin if your doctor approves.

- Camps in Massachusetts for Children with Diabetes
  Eliot P. Joslin Camp for Boys
  Charlton, MA

- Clara Barton Camp for Girls
  North Oxford, MA 01537

- Contact the Joslin Diabetes Foundation, 1 Joslin Place,
  Boston, MA 02215
  1-617-732-2646/1-508-757-1211 (winter)/1-508-987-2056
  (summer)

- Information on other camps can be obtained from the
  local chapters of the American Diabetes Association or
  the Juvenile Diabetes Foundation.

Years 12 Through 17

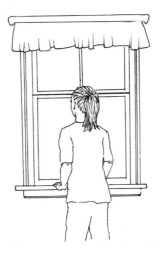

At adolescence, your child will greatly resent dependence
on a parent. Once you **and** your child are educated about
diabetes, he or she must be permitted to participate in
treatment decisions. Adolescents may act as if they do not
have diabetes, ignoring their treatments (especially diet)
and falsifying blood sugar tests. They may also need to see
for themselves just how awful they can feel before accepting the importance of control. Depression in adolescents
with diabetes is not uncommon. They are aware of diabetic
complications and death. They wish to be carefree and
often refuse to adhere to their regimen because they assume that they will die young. Listen to your children

express fears and problems. Sometimes they need to vent, and sometimes they need help. Make sure that your child understands the importance of good control—significant improvements in diabetes treatment are likely during his or her lifetime (see Chapter 15)—and make sure your child is aware of the many people with diabetes who lead full, rich lives. Don't hesitate to contact a professional counselor. Specialized psychologists are available to help with children who have diabetes.

Sports and Gym Class

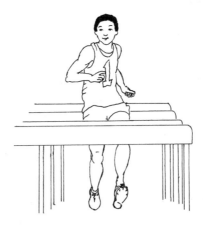

Diabetes is no reason for missing out on sports or skipping gym class. In fact, exercise is an important factor in diabetes control. If your child has gym class before lunch, increase the morning snack of carbohydrates and protein. If your child participates in after-school sports, increase the afternoon snack. Make sure that your child understands that he or she must always carry fast-acting sugar. It won't do any good in a gym locker. Also make sure that the coach and a few friends know how to help in case of a reaction.

Groups and camps for teens with diabetes can help by offering them a chance to share their troubles and concerns with peers. Teenagers need someone to talk with besides their parents. Let your teenager meet with his or her healthcare provider alone.

At the end of adolescence, around 19 to 20 years, your child will begin to mature in attitude and responsibility. Democratic guidance is the best approach as children progress from dependence to independence. Set realistic limits and goals, and use positive reinforcement. Praise is more helpful than punishments and threats.

School

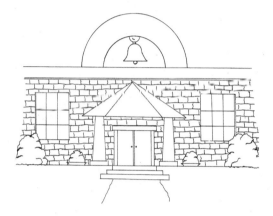

Teachers, school nurses, and other school personnel need to understand your child's condition. Part III contains a concise overview of diabetes that will help school personnel cope with your child's special needs.

- Make a photocopy of Part III and bring those pages to your child's school nurse or teacher at the beginning of each school year. Your child's teacher will also benefit from specific information about your child's particular diabetes control requirements.

- Fill in a copy of the form on page 216 and give it to your child's teacher at the beginning of each school year.

- Be prepared to answer any other questions that the teacher might have about your child's special needs.

- Use copies of the form on page 217 to communicate your child's daily blood glucose testing and dietary requirements.

- It's also a good idea to visit or call the school about once a month to see how things are going.

Baby Sitters

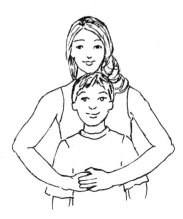

Like any parent, you deserve a night out once in a while. Don't let your fear of leaving your child with someone who does not understand diabetes keep you from enjoying life. For your own piece of mind, instruct your trusted baby sitter or relative in the basics of diabetes care. Include the following:

- A brief overview of diabetes.

- Blood sugar testing instructions.

- Insulin injection instructions.

- Appropriate snacks and meals.

- Warning signs and treatment of low blood sugar.

Keep supplies, equipment, snacks, and quick sugar food all together in a special location. Prepare a checklist that specifies what needs to be done at what time and written instructions for emergency procedures.

Make sure the baby sitter knows how to reach you **and** your child's healthcare provider at all times. Make photocopies of the forms in the following section, or design your own.

To the Baby Sitter

_____ has diabetes.

- Diabetes means that this child's pancreas does not make enough insulin. Without insulin, food cannot be used properly. A child with diabetes must take daily injections of insulin and must balance his or her food and exercise.
- An insulin reaction may occur if the blood sugar gets too low—especially before meals or after exercise.

Warning Signs of Insulin Reactions

- Paleness
- Perspiration
- Shakiness, nervousness
- Headache, nausea, stomachache
- Changes of mood
- Confusion
- Irritability
- Our child usually behaves as follows when having a reaction:

_____

_____

If this happens, immediately give the child sugar in the form of:

- Glucose gel or tablets **or** _____
- Syrup, 2 tablespoons **or** _____
- Fruit juice, 1/2 cup **or** _____
- Soft drink (**not** diet or sugar free), cup **or** _____
- 10 jelly beans **or** _____
- You will find this supply of sugar: _____

_____

_____

- Repeat this feeding if the child does not improve in 10 to 15 minutes.
- Follow with a milk and cookie or sandwich snack.
- If the child does not improve after eating the snack, call the parents or physician.

Part III: What School Personnel Should Know About the Student with Diabetes

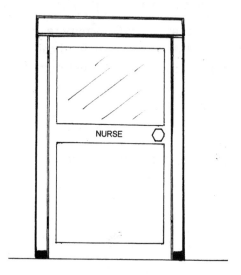

The American Diabetes Association Committee on Diabetes in Youth prepared this information, and the National Education Association Department of School Nurses endorsed it. We encourage you to print out these pages and bring them to your child's teacher every year.

General Information

All school personnel (teachers, nurses, principals, lunch-room workers, playground and hall supervisors, bus drivers, counselors, etc.) must be informed that a student has diabetes. It is imperative that all personnel understand the fundamentals of the disease and its care.

Diabetes is not an infectious disease. It results from failure of the pancreas to make a sufficient amount of insulin. Without insulin, food cannot be used properly. Diabetes currently cannot be cured, but it can be controlled. Treatment consists of daily injections of insulin and a prescribed food plan. Children with diabetes can participate in all school activities and should not be considered different from other students. It is essential that school personnel have conferences with parents early in each school year to obtain more specific information about the individual child and his or her specific needs. Communication and cooperation between parents and school personnel can help the diabetic child have a happy and well-adjusted school experience.

Insulin Reactions

Insulin reactions occur when the amount of sugar in the blood is too low. This is caused by an imbalance of insulin, too much exercise, or too little food. Under these circumstances, the body sends out numerous warning signs. If these signs are recognized early, reactions may be promptly terminated by giving some form of sugar. If a reaction is not treated, unconsciousness and convulsions may result. The child may recognize some of the following warning signs of low blood sugar and should be encouraged to report them.

Warning Signs of an Insulin Reaction

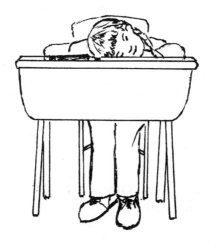

- Excessive hunger
- Blurred vision
- Poor coordination
- Perspiration
- Irritability
- Abdominal pain or nausea
- Pallor
- Crying
- Dizziness
- Inability to concentrate
- Inappropriate actions/responses
- Nervousness or trembling
- Drowsiness or fatigue

Treatment

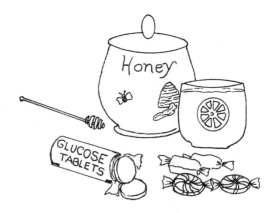

At the first sign of any of these warning signs, give sugar immediately in one of the following forms:

- Glucose tablets or gel.
- Fruit juice, 0.5 cup.
- Carbonated beverage (not diet or sugarless soda), 6 ounces.
- Ten jelly beans or soft candy.
- A sugar that the parent has provided.

A student who is experiencing a reaction may need coaxing to eat. If improvement does not occur within

15 to 20 minutes, repeat the feeding. If the child does not improve after administration of the second feeding containing sugar, the parents or a physician should be called. When the child improves, he or she should be given a small feeding of a half sandwich and a glass of milk. He or she should then resume normal school activities, and the parents should be advised of the incident.

Children with diabetes follow a prescribed diet and may select their foods from the school lunch menu or bring their own lunch. Lunchroom managers should be made aware of the child's dietary needs, which may include mid-morning and midafternoon snacks to help avoid insulin reactions. Adequate time should be provided for finishing meals.

Blood sugar testing may need to be done during the school day. This information is needed to determine an appropriate diet/insulin/exercise plan. It may also be helpful to get a blood sugar test if the child becomes ill during the day.

General Advice

The child with diabetes should be carefully observed in class, particularly before lunch. It is best not to schedule physical education just before lunch; if possible, the child should not be assigned to a late lunch period. Many children require nourishment before strenuous exercise. Teachers and nurses should have sugar available at all times. The child with diabetes should also carry a sugar supply and be permitted to treat a reaction when it occurs.

Diabetic coma, a serious complication of the disease, results from uncontrolled diabetes. This does not come on suddenly and generally does not need to be a concern to school personnel.

Teacher Information

Child's Name _____ Date _____

Parent's Name _____

Address _____

Phone (home) _____ (work) _____

Alternate person to call in emergency _____

Relationship _____ Daytime Phone _____

Physician's Name _____

Address _____

Phone _____

Signs and symptoms the child usually exhibits preceding insulin reaction:

_____

_____

_____

Time of day reaction most likely to occur: _____

Most effective treatment (sweets most readily accepted):

_____

_____

Morning or afternoon snack: _____

_____

Suggested "treats" for in-school parties: _____

_____

Note: A child with diabetes may need to check his/her blood sugar during the day to find out about his or her blood sugar level. The parents will show you the method that they use and give you guidelines about when to notify them. Children usually are able to do their own blood glucose testing.

Notes for Today

Child's Name _____

Teacher _____

Test blood sugar at:

_____   _____   _____

And record below:

_____   _____   _____

Serve: _____

_____

_____

_____ at _____o'clock

Serve: _____

_____

_____

_____ at _____o'clock

Serve: _____

_____

_____

_____ at _____o'clock

Parents are at:

_____ (Phone) _____

Physician:

_____ (Phone) _____

Part IV: How to Support a Family Member

Support is an essential part of good diabetes care. When a family member or a close friend has diabetes, he or she will need your support. Diabetes can affect every area of family life. Support can come in many ways, and needs can change over time.

To be successful in helping your family member with diabetes, follow these steps:

- Learn all about diabetes, the treatment plan, and hypoglycemia.

- Express your feelings, worries, and fears.

- Be realistic about how closely he or she will follow their diabetes plan.

- Don't be pushy or try to control the person's behavior.

Helpful Hints

- Ask how you can help.

- Ask how a person feels when an insulin reaction happens.

- Take walks together.

- Shop for groceries together and decide on some healthy meals and snacks.

- Think of cues that may help the person remember his or her medication.

- Be aware of the frustrations of maintaining diabetic control.

- Follow healthy habits yourself.

- If appropriate, take an interest in blood sugar test results.

- Express concern for his or her health.

Things Not to Do

- Be the "diabetic police."
- Argue about what is allowed.
- Nag or be pushy or yell.
- Threaten.
- Ignore your own health.
- Smoke.
- Allow them to be repeatedly abusive under the guise of hypoglycemia.

Further Reading

This book is for clinicians, but may be helpful:

The Art of Empowerment. Bob Anderson, EdD, and Martha Funnell, MS, RN, CDE.

CHAPTER 14

Traveling

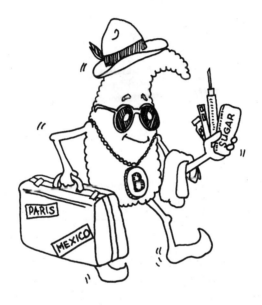

Whether you travel for business or pleasure, diabetes travels with you. You can't ignore your diet, exercise, and medications or your insulin regimen when you're away from home. Your diabetes should not cause you to feel trapped. You can go anywhere a person without diabetes can—just remember these simple tips to make traveling a lot easier.

Diabetes may be a constant in your life, but don't let it trap you. With a few simple precautions, you can travel anywhere.

For All People with Diabetes

Make a Diabetes Supply Checklist Before You Leave

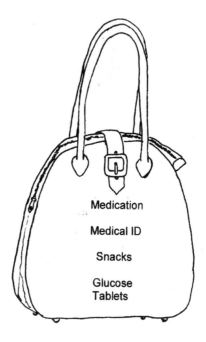

Medication

Medical ID

Snacks

Glucose
Tablets

- Have a medical checkup. If you are going to an area where diarrhea might be a problem, ask your healthcare provider to prescribe an antidiarrhea medication. You may also want to take along something to prevent or treat nausea.

- Carry some form of diabetes identification with you stating that you have diabetes (a bracelet, wallet card, or necklace).

- Take extra insulin and syringes, and if you use an insulin pump, take double infusion sets and reservoirs.

- Carry snacks to be prepared for delays and changes.

- You'll be asking for trouble if you take new shoes. Leave them at home.

- Food may be quite different. Spend some time learning how to select food from what is available.

- Have required vaccinations weeks ahead of your departure time to avoid reactions that may disturb your blood sugar balance while away from home.

- When planning a trip to areas where English is not typical, try to learn how to say this in the necessary language: "I have diabetes; please get me to a doctor" or "sugar or juice, please."

- Choose hotels carefully. Know what facilities are offered and what services are available.

- Always wear or carry some form of medical identification. A tag, bracelet, or necklace with the medical emblem is best.

- If you take oral medications for diabetes, carry enough for the entire trip. You may have trouble getting your prescription filled in a foreign country.

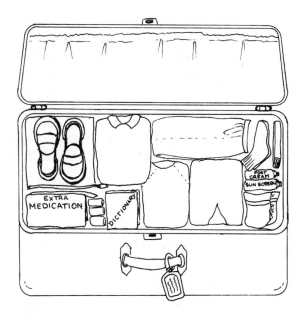

- Take along familiar blood sugar equipment and extra test strips. Remember, many changes take place during travel, and the only way to assess your control is by frequent monitoring.

- For a list of English-speaking doctors in other countries, contact the International Association for Medical Assistance to Travelers, 417 Center Street, Lewiston, New York 14092.

While Traveling

- If you are traveling by plane, notify the airline 24 hours in advance if you want a special meal. **Carry all medications with you on the plane.** Syringes, lancets, meters, and pumps are only allowed on the plane if you have an unopened vial of insulin in the box with the pharmacy label on it **or** diabetes pills that are in the original bottle with a pharmacy label on it.

- Stay as close to your routine mealtime and medication time as possible.

- Keep active while in transit. If you are traveling by car, stop every so often and take a walk for at least 5 minutes. On a train, walk through the cars now and then. On a bus, take advantage of stopovers by getting out and walking around to stretch cramped muscles. While sitting on a plane, try to get up as often as you can and walk every 1 to 2 hours. Move and stretch your feet and legs often.

- On car trips, carry food in case of an emergency. A cell phone can be a plus. A flat tire or mechanical failure may leave you stranded far from a restaurant at your scheduled mealtime.

- Drink extra water.

At Your Destination

- Cruise ships are delightful. They offer a great selection of foods, but often too much! You don't have to clean your plate. Ships have tracks to walk on and usually an exercise room; thus, there's no excuse for gaining weight.

- You can eat anywhere, but full-service restaurants are usually more compatible with your need for a balanced diet. Don't wait until the last minute to order from room service. Order at least 30 minutes before your scheduled mealtime.

- In South or Central America, Asia, and Africa, avoid the following foods: raw meats, milk, ice cream, cream sauces, soft cheese, water or ice cubes, peeled fruits, and lettuce and other leafy vegetables.

- Always carry small cans of juice, dried fruit, peanut butter, crackers, or packaged cheese and crackers, which can be a substitute meal if necessary.

- Don't overexpose your skin the first few days you spend in the sun. Apply SPF 15 or higher sunscreen to protect against burning.

- Remember your basic rules of foot care (see Chapter 11). Don't wear new shoes on vacation. Check your feet daily. If you get blisters from walking, apply a mild antiseptic and a small gauze pad held in place with nonallergic tape. Don't break blisters!

- Don't walk barefoot on hot beach sand or in areas where seashells may cut your skin. Always wear beach or swim shoes, sandals, or some other foot covering.

- If you are ill during a trip, remember your rules for sick day management (see Chapter 10). Check blood sugar frequently. Ice chips or sips of regular (not diet) cola or ginger ale are good for nausea. Try to take some every hour. You may also try cereal, milk, ice cream, tea, toast, broth, and soups to replace full meals. If you take oral medications for diabetes and you are too sick to eat, try to drink plenty of liquids. If your blood sugars remain high, call for help.

For People Requiring Insulin

- Carry insulin and syringes with you. **Insulin does not need to be refrigerated,** but you must protect it from extreme heat or cold. Do not leave your insulin on the dashboard of a hot car. If traveling by plane, have insulin in your carry-on luggage.

- Carry a letter from your doctor stating that you have diabetes and must carry insulin syringes and monitoring equipment with you. This will protect you in case of any questions about your syringes or in case you lose them and need replacements.

- Always carry fast-acting sugar.

- You may need to adjust insulin or food according to your activity level. Bike riding, hiking, and walking tours burn up a lot of calories. To be safe, check your blood sugar frequently.

- Make sure that traveling companions know the signs of an insulin reaction and how to help you with fast-acting sugars.

- Test more frequently when on vacation. No vacation is free from diabetes.

- It's easy to gain weight on vacation; thus, taste new foods, but remember portion control.

- Walking tours burn a lot of calories. Be sure to carry snacks, sugar, and water.

- Stop and rest as often as you need. Remember that this is a vacation and should be fun!

For People on Insulin Traveling Across Time Zones

- When planning a trip that will take you across time zones, consult your healthcare provider about adjusting your meals and insulin/medication schedules. On a long plane trip across time zones, keep your watch at point-of-departure time and take snacks and meals accordingly. Resume normal doses the next day at point-of-arrival time.

Guidelines for Crossing Time Zones

Heading East (Shorter Day) Less Insulin	
West →	→ East
8 a.m.	6–10 p.m. Point of departure time
Take 2/3-dose of intermediate or long-acting insulin	Take 2/3-dose of intermediate or long-acting insulin

Take your usual (or adjusted) dose of Humalog, Novolog, or regular insulin. The next morning, take usual, full doses of insulin. Set your watch to the new time.

Heading West (Longer Day) More Insulin		
East →	→	→ West
8 a.m.	6–8 p.m. Point of departure time	6–10 p.m. Point of arrival time
Take the usual dose of intermediate or long-acting insulin plus usual dose of regular insulin	Take an extra dose of Humalog, Novolog, or regular ____units if indicated by blood sugar of ____ mg	Take a usual dose of intermediate or long-acting insulin

Resources

The Diabetes Travel Guide. Davida F. Kreiger, MSN, RN, CS, CDE.

Traveler's Hotline:
1-877-FYI-TRIP
www.cdc.gov/travel
International Society of Travel Medicine
1-770-736-7060
www.istem.org

CHAPTER 15

Diabetes Research

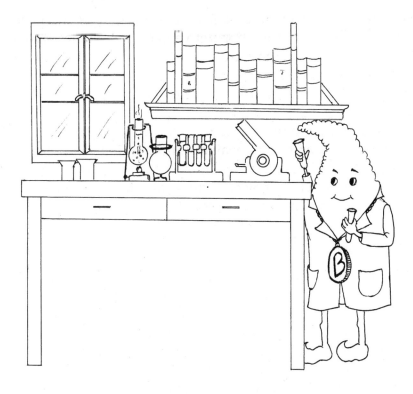

At present, diabetes has no easy cure. However, researchers have begun promising and exciting studies into finding ways of preventing, treating, and curing diabetes.

The ultimate goals for diabetes research are to:

1. Cure the disease.

2. Prevent the disease from occurring.

3. Prevent complications and find better treatments.

Curing Diabetes

At present, the only cure for diabetes is to replace the beta cells (insulin producing cells). The principal methods that researchers are investigating include:

- Pancreas transplantation: Pancreas transplants are most often done in conjunction with a necessary kidney transplant. Following the transplant, the patient receives powerful immunosuppressive drugs to prevent rejection. These drugs prevent the immune system from destroying the foreign tissue, such as the new kidney or pancreas. Because the immune system normally protects against infections and guards against cancer, immunosuppressive drugs make the recipient susceptible to infections and cancer. These powerful drugs also have side effects that can damage normal tissues.

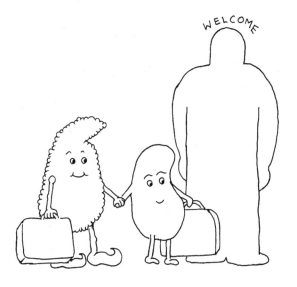

- Islet transplantation: Islet transplants have received considerable attention from diabetes researchers. The treatment involves injecting islets (beta cells) so that they lodge in the liver. The procedure consists of obtaining the pancreas from a deceased donor and isolating the islets from this pancreas. Then the islets (about a tablespoon) are infused into a large vein that empties into the liver, called the portal vein, while the patient is under local anesthesia. At present, immunosuppressive medications are still needed to prevent rejection of the transplanted islets.

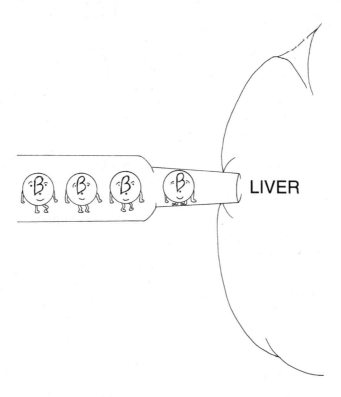

LIVER

Other current research endeavors include:

- Encapsulated islets: Researchers have attempted to encase beta cells in porous material to prevent them from rejection. The goal is to design a protection that does not allow the immune cells to enter and destroy the beta cells, but does allow insulin produced by the beta cells to pass out of the protective capsule.

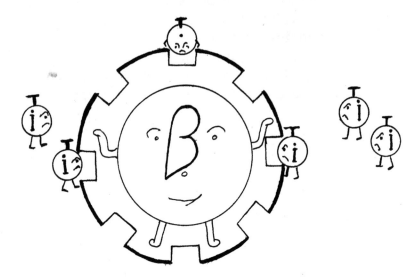

- Tolerance induction: "Tolerance" is a term to describe the transplantation of a foreign tissue without the continuous use of immunosuppressive drugs. Various strategies are being pursued to permit the islets to be accepted by the recipients' immune system.

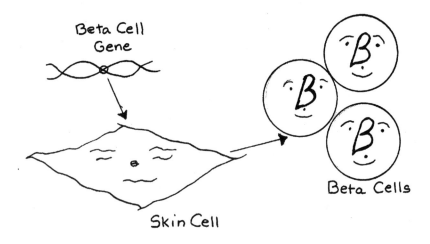

Beta Cell Gene

Beta Cells

Skin Cell

- Creating beta cells: This concept involves genetic manipulation of normal cells (e.g., skin cells) to introduce the genes that produce insulin. These genes would then create bioengineered beta cells in the body.

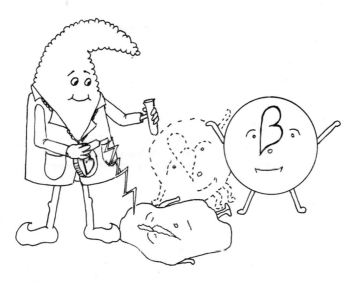

- Regenerating beta cells: Because removal of part of the liver causes liver tissue to regenerate itself, scientists are seeking a similar process for beta cells. Scientists are also studying the signals that are necessary to make beta cells during normal fetal development and attempting to repeat this process in the adult.

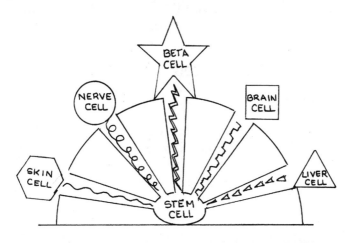

- Stem cells: Stem cells have the ability to make new cells, including beta cells. Scientists are isolating stem cells and using various substances to encourage them to become new beta cells.

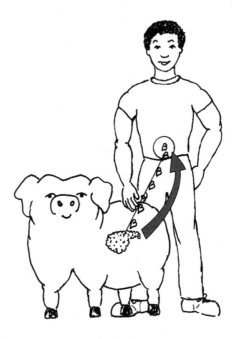

- Xenograft: Beta cells from other animals produce insulin that can work in humans. The use of beta cells from pigs is also an alternative source for human cells. A major problem with this treatment relates to the possible transmission of infections from animals to humans.

Prevention of Diabetes

Type 1 Diabetes

The current strategy to prevent the disease from occurring depends on identifying the factors that start the disease in the first place.

Certain genes in the immune system appear to make a person susceptible to diabetes. These genes make the immune system attack and destroy beta cells. The genes involved are called Human Leukocyte Antigens (HLA). People who have the genes HLA DR3 and HLA DR4 are susceptible to Type 1 diabetes.

Immune System

Although the genes make you susceptible to Type 1 diabetes, they are not the only factor. In order to get Type 1 diabetes, your immune system must become destructive. Most scientists believe that many people have immune cells that are able to destroy beta cells (autoreactive lymphocytes), but that these immune cells are kept in balance by other immune cells (regulatory lymphocytes) that limit the attacks on beta cells.

An imbalance of these immune cells can be observed in the earliest stages of diabetes by measuring the presence of cells called autoantibodies in blood samples. Autoantibodies are antibodies that are directed against oneself. People with a high number of these autoantibodies have a high probability of becoming diabetic.

Immunosuppressive drugs have been used in an attempt to stop the immune system from destroying its own beta cells. Although the drugs do halt beta cell destruction, their long-term use is impossible because of side effects. Once the drugs are stopped, beta cell destruction resumes. Researchers are looking for ways to prevent this destruction by looking for more selective immune drugs as well as strategies to increase the number of regulatory cells.

Once all of the pieces of the puzzle are identified, it may be possible to develop safe strategies for preventing Type 1 diabetes.

Type 2 Diabetes

Distinct, abnormal genes are involved in Type 2 diabetes. Abnormalities have been found in both the genes that signal the beta cell to release insulin and the genes that make insulin respond.

Many of these genes may be abnormal at birth, but the abnormalities might go unnoticed because the body's cells can sometimes compensate. However, under stressful conditions, the cells no longer can work properly. For example, obesity, pregnancy, emotional stress, and certain medications can tip the balance so that the beta cells can no longer keep up with the demand. In the future, we will be able to identify specific gene abnormalities and provide specific treatment to cure the disease.

Prevention of Complications and Better Treatments

Many new strategies for prevention of diabetes complications are available or are being researched. Likewise, improvements in diabetes treatment are coming at a fast pace. The table that follows lists many of them.

Present	Under Investigation	Future
Better Treatment:		
New types of insulin with different actions	Oral insulin Nasal insulin Inhaled insulin Insulin patch	Oral pills that will act like insulin
Monitoring		
Glucose monitoring	Gluco-Watch	Non-invasive monitors
Oral antidiabetogenic agents	More specific oral agents Appetite suppressants	Genetic defect and specific treatment
COMPLICATIONS:		
Kidney		
Blood pressure lowering agents (use of ACE inhibitor medications)	More specific oral drugs with less side-effects	Genetics that cause the kidney damage and blood pressure elevation and specific treatment
Nerves		
Pain relief	Drugs that block the glucose from destroying the nerves	Genetics involved in nerve destruction and specific treatment
Eyes		
Laser RX	Drugs that block the new vessels that cause blindness	Genetics of the defect and to selectively stop them from occurring
Heart/Blood vessels		
Treatment of blood pressure. Cholesterol lowering agents Low-dose aspirin Angioplasty, coronary artery bypass surgery	Drugs and treatment to block some of the production of atherosclerosis	Genetics and to stop factors that make atherosclerosis Make new blood vessels (use stem cells) Reverse atherosclerosis

Although some of the ideas in this chapter may seem remote or improbable, cure and prevention of diabetes are certainly not impossible goals. No one knows what the future may bring. Research offers hope. Hope for a cure, hope for prevention of diabetes, and hope for prevention of complications and better treatments. Your job at the present time is to maintain good control until our hope is a reality.

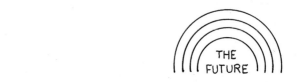

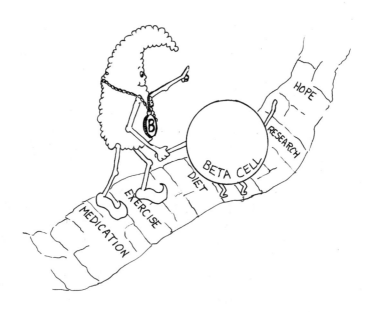

Glossary

Acetone: Chemical substance produced during breakdown of body fat (ketones).

Acidosis: Abnormal state; too much acid in the blood. Can be a serious complication of Type 1 diabetes.

Aerobic exercise: Exercise that uses increased oxygen and stimulates heart and lung activity.

Albumin: Blood protein that may appear in urine when kidneys are damaged.

Alpha cells: Glucagon-producing cells of the islets of Langerhans.

Alpha-glucosidase inhibitors: Oral antidiabetic drug that inhibits the absorption of sugar from the gut.

Amino acids: Individual food units that combine to make proteins.

Anaerobic exercise: Exercise that requires no increase in oxygen demand; usually strength training activity.

Arteriosclerosis: Thickening and rigidification of artery walls.

Atherosclerosis: Thickening of artery walls from fatty deposits.

Artificial pancreas: A device that releases insulin in response to blood sugar demands (in research).

Aspart: Rapid-acting insulin (Novolog).

Athlete's foot: Fungus infection of feet.

Basal insulin: Steady available pulsed flow of insulin.

Beta cells: Insulin-producing cells of the islets of Langerhans.

Biguanides: Oral antidiabetic drug that inhibits glucose production by the liver.

BMI: Body Mass Index, a method to quantify body fat based on height and weight.

Bolus insulin: Burst of insulin delivered with meals or to correct a high blood sugar.

Callus: Hard skin thickening due to friction or pressure.

Calorie: Unit used to express heat or energy value of food.

Carbohydrate counting: A method of counting grams or portions of carbohydrates consumed at meals and snacks.

Carbohydrate: One of three major food substances (examples: sugar, starch).

Cataract: Clouding of lens of eye.

Cell: Unit of body structure.

Cholesterol: Fatty substance normally present in blood.

Claudication: Pains in calf muscles due to decrease in blood supply.

Coma: Loss of consciousness.

Coping skills: Behaviors that modify stress.

Coronary insufficiency: Impaired blood supply to heart.

Correction factor: The points of blood sugar that are lowered by one unit of insulin.

Crystalline insulin: Regular insulin.

Cystitis: Inflammation of the urinary bladder.

Diabetes complications: Adverse effects of long-term high blood sugar and genetics.

Diabetes educator: Nurse, physician, or dietitian who has extensive knowledge of diabetes and teaching/learning skills.

Diabetes self-management: Ability to take responsibility for one's own diabetes control.

Dietitian: A professional who advises people with special health needs on the types and amounts of foods to eat.

Fat: One of three major food substances (examples: butter, cream).

Fiber: Indigestible part of fruits, vegetables, cereals, and grains.

Food exchange: Foods grouped together due to similarities in nutritional value.

Fructose: Carbohydrate sugar found in fruits and candy.

Gangrene: Death of tissue, usually due to loss of blood supply.

Gestational diabetes: Diabetes that is diagnosed during pregnancy.

Glargine: Long-acting insulin.

Glomerulus: Microscopic part of kidney that filters blood.

Glucagon: Hormone produced by alpha cells to release glycogen stored in liver and muscles. Glucagon injections are used to treat serious insulin reactions in persons with diabetes.

Glucose tolerance test: Test for detecting diabetes.

Glucose: Basic sugar used to fuel body cells.

Glycogen: Form in which most carbohydrates are stored in the body.

Glycosuria: Sugar in urine.

Gram: Metric unit of weight.

HDL: High-density lipoprotein; "good cholesterol."

Hemoglobin A1c: A blood test that measures a person's average blood glucose over the past 2–3 months.

Heredity: Inheritance of traits from ancestors; a major cause of diabetes.

Hormone: Chemical substance produced in body glands and circulated in blood.

Hyperglycemia: High concentration of sugar in blood (hyper = high).

Hypoglycemia: Low concentration of sugar in blood (hypo = low).

Hypoglycemia unawareness: Loss of catecholamine response (sweating and shaking) to hypoglycemia.

Impotence: Inability to sustain an erection.

Insulin pump: Computerized device that delivers insulin by basal mode and bolus doses.

Insulin reaction: Release of certain hormones (catecholamines) in response to hypoglycemia. The hormones cause sweating and shaking.

Insulin resistance: A condition that opposes the action of insulin in the body.

Insulin sensitivity factor: A calculated ratio giving the number of points of blood sugar lowered by 1 unit of insulin (used interchangeably with "correction factor").

Insulin-to-carbohydrate ratio: A calculated ratio giving the number of carbohydrates covered by 1 unit of insulin.

Insulin: Hormone produced by beta cells to facilitate entry of glucose into body cells.

Islet cell transplant: Placing donor islets into a recipient with diabetes to "cure" diabetes.

Islets of Langerhans: Clusters of alpha, beta, delta, and polypeptide cells throughout the pancreas.

Ketonuria: Ketone in urine.

Keto-Stix: Test for ketone (acetone) in urine.

Kidney threshold: Level at which sugar "spills" over into urine.

Kussmaul breathing: Deep, rapid breathing seen in diabetic acidosis.

Lactose: Milk sugar.

LDL: Low-density lipoprotein; "bad cholesterol."

Lente insulin: Intermediate-acting insulin.

Lispro: Rapid-acting insulin (Humalog).

Macrovascular disease: Arteriosclerotic and atherosclerotic changes in larger blood vessels.

Meal plan: Individualized guideline for meals and snacks.

Metabolism: Conversion of food substances to energy.

Monilia: Fungus infection (*candida*) common in diabetes, frequently in the vagina.

Monitoring blood glucose: Periodic testing of one's blood sugar by obtaining a small drop of blood, applying to a test strip, and reading the result on a meter.

Nephropathy: Degenerative kidney disease that may occur in long-term diabetes.

Neuropathy: Disorder of nerves causing loss of sensation and reflexes and/or burning or stabbing pain, especially at night.

NPH insulin: Intermediate-acting insulin.

Obesity: BMI of 30 kg/m^2 or more.

Oral antidiabetic agents: Oral drugs that increase the effectiveness of insulin.

Oral hypoglycemia agents: Oral drugs that lower blood sugar by increasing insulin and/or increasing insulin effectiveness.

Overweight: BMI of 25 to 29.9% kg/m^2.

Pancreas: Gland deep in abdomen, behind stomach, that produces hormones (insulin, glucagon) and digestive enzymes.

Polydipsia: Excessive thirst.

Polyphagia: Excessive hunger.

Polyuria: Excessive urination.

Post-prandial: After a meal.

Protein: One of the three major food substances; food used to build body tissues.

Pruritus: Itching.

Regular insulin: Fast-acting insulin.

Retinopathy: Disorders of retina (nerve tissue in the eye) seen in diabetes.

Saccharin: Artificial sweetener.

Semi-lente insulin: Rapid-acting insulin.

Sorbitol: Artificial sweetener.

Sucrose: Ordinary table sugar; breaks down to glucose and fructose.

Sulfonylureas: Oral hypoglycemic drug.

Target blood sugar: Goal for blood sugar level.

Thiazolidinediones: Oral antidiabetic drug that reduces insulin resistance.

Triglycerides: Type of blood fat.

Ultralente insulin: Long-acting insulin.

Index

Insulin reaction: 116, 129, 132–140,
    213–215
Insulin resistance: 53
Insurance: 35–36, 66–67
Intensive insulin therapy
    Carbohydrate counting and: 96
    Hypoglycemia unawareness: 136
    Introduction to: 147–152
    Meal flexibility and: 47–49
    Self-monitoring of blood glucose
        (SMBG): 62
International Association for
    Medical Assistance to
    Travelers: 224
International Society of Travel
    Medicine: 227
Intestinal disease: 159
Islets of Langerhans: 8–9
Islet transplants: 231

J

Job discrimination: 34–35
Joslin Diabetes Foundation: 207
Juvenile diabetes: See Type 1
    diabetes
Juvenile Diabetes Foundation
    International: 24

K

Ketoacidosis, diabetic: 44, 170
Ketones: 17, 43, 68, 162–163
Ketonuria: 17
Kidney disease: 158, 188–190
Kidney threshold: 14–15

L

Labels, reading of for meal plans:
    84–85
Laboratory tests, and fasting: 60
Lancets: 131
Leg cramps, at night: 17
Lente insulin: 120–122
Lipoatrophy: 129
Lipohypertrophy: 129
Lispro insulin: 120–122
Liver, and glycogen storage: 7–8,
    10–12, 53, 139
Liver disease: 158, 159
Logs, for recording blood sugar
    levels: 72–74
Low-calorie foods: 89
Low-density lipoprotein (bad
    cholesterol): 87
Low-fat foods: 89

M

Macrovascular disease: 192–196
Magnifiers: 131
Management of diabetes: See Self-
    management of diabetes
Meal plans (See also Nutrition)
    Alcoholic drinks: 89–90
    Behavior, changing of: 92–93
    Carbohydrate counting: 80–81,
        94–96
    Eating out: 90–91
    Exchange plan: 81–82
    Fiber: 88
    Food pyramid: 82–83
    Need for: 79–80
    Oral medications and: 59
    Plate method: 83–84
    Reading labels: 84–85
    Self-monitoring of blood glucose
        (SMBG): 62–63
    Sick day and: 166–167
    Sweets: 89
    Type 1 diabetes: 45, 47–49
    Weight loss guidelines: 86–89
Medicare: 36
Medications (See also Oral
    medications for diabetes)
    Diabetes factor: 21, 53
    Hypoglycemia unawareness:
        137–138
    Interactions of: 37–38, 157
    Nonprescription medicines: 37–38,
        168–170
Medigap: 36
Medtronic MiniMed, Inc.: 70, 153
Metabolic cataracts: 185
Meters, for SMBG: 66–67, 71
Monitoring: 68–71 (See also Self-
    monitoring of blood glucose
    (SMBG))
Monounsaturated fat: 87
Mumps: 42

N

Nail fungi: 179
National Diabetes Information
    Clearing House: 24
Native Americans, and diabetes: 54
Nausea: 168, 191
Needles: 130–132
Nephropathy: 188–190
Nerve damage: 172–173, 190–192
Neuroglycopenia: 134
Neuropathy: 172–173, 190–192
Night leg cramps: 17